Medicine in the Middle Ages

Medicine in the Middle Ages

Surviving the Times

Juliana Cummings

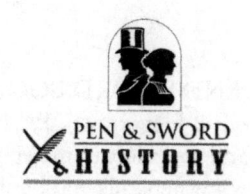

PEN & SWORD
HISTORY

First published in Great Britain in 2021 by
Pen & Sword History
An imprint of
Pen & Sword Books Ltd
Yorkshire – Philadelphia

Copyright © Juliana Cummings 2021

ISBN 978 1 52677 934 2

The right of Juliana Cummings to be identified as Author of this work has been asserted by her in accordance with the Copyright, Designs and Patents Act 1988.

A CIP catalogue record for this book is
available from the British Library.

All rights reserved. No part of this book may be reproduced or transmitted in any form or by any means, electronic or mechanical including photocopying, recording or by any information storage and retrieval system, without permission from the Publisher in writing.

Printed and bound in the UK by CPI Group (UK) Ltd,
Croydon, CR0 4YY.

Pen & Sword Books Limited incorporates the imprints of Atlas, Archaeology, Aviation, Discovery, Family History, Fiction, History, Maritime, Military, Military Classics, Politics, Select, Transport, True Crime, Air World, Frontline Publishing, Leo Cooper, Remember When, Seaforth Publishing, The Praetorian Press, Wharncliffe Local History, Wharncliffe Transport, Wharncliffe True Crime and White Owl.

For a complete list of Pen & Sword titles please contact

PEN & SWORD BOOKS LIMITED
47 Church Street, Barnsley, South Yorkshire, S70 2AS, England
E-mail: enquiries@pen-and-sword.co.uk
Website: www.pen-and-sword.co.uk

Or

PEN AND SWORD BOOKS
1950 Lawrence Rd, Havertown, PA 19083, USA
E-mail: Uspen-and-sword@casematepublishers.com
Website: www.penandswordbooks.com

Contents

Acknowledgments		vi
Introduction		viii
Chapter 1	A Foundation for Western Medicine is Built	1
Chapter 2	The Influence of Christianity Spreads	13
Chapter 3	A Hierarchy of Importance	23
Chapter 4	The Spreading of Disease	41
Chapter 5	A Woman's Duty	68
Chapter 6	The Role of the Caretaker	94
Chapter 7	Medicine on the Battlefield	125
Chapter 8	Housing the Poor, the Sick and the Insane	140
Chapter 9	A Culture of Death	166
Notes and Sources		189
Bibliography		193

Acknowledgments

I want to thank my husband, my parents, and my sister for their continued support in all my writing endeavours. Thank you to my dog, Pumpkin, for keeping me company while I wrote for what seemed like endless hours. Thank you to my cousin, Bryan, for making me look like a big star when I'm really not.

Brenda, my dear friend, thank you for your continued support and willingness to read everything I threw at you. Thank you to my dear friend, Jane, for being my own personal cheerleader. I can always count on you as a proper mate.

It's easy to write historical fiction, as it's essentially your interpretation of the story. Though it takes research, it's not nearly as much as it takes to write non-fiction. So, I want to thank all of the other history nerds, like myself, for your plethora of information that was so valuable to my cause. Your blogs and documentaries, and lectures offered me so much insight into the world of medieval medicine. Professor Carole Rawcliffe, your talks on leprosy were indispensable, and I got so much pleasure out of listening to you.

Thank you to Professor Lorraine Attreed at Holy Cross College for everything you did to help me start this journey. You offered an endless supply of materials and information essential for this book, and I'm so honoured to call you my friend. Thank you for taking the time to visit with me and "Talk Tudor" and for always returning my emails right away. Your insightful and learned help was always what I needed. Your encouragement and support for my book were valued more than you know. Your expertise in English medieval history is used far beyond what you teach in the classroom. It is much appreciated. I'm glad to have known you for almost twenty-five years!

Thank you to historian Matt Lewis for being kind enough to let me post a guest blog on your website years ago. I reached out to you as a fellow writer and avid fan of your work. Little did I know, you would take the time to respond with as much support as you did. If not for that, Pen & Sword may have never reached out to me. So, thank you for taking a chance on me even though I was a Henry VIII fan! And thank you for assuring me that, yes, Pen & Sword was the real deal. I am eternally grateful.

And finally, thank you to all of the staff at Pen & Sword for making this possible. Eleri Pipien, thank you for reaching out to me. Getting your email asking if I was interested in writing a book didn't seem real at the time! Thank you to Claire Hopkins for your unwavering support for my work and your reassurance with any questions I had. Sarah-Beth Watkins, thank you for your kindness and patience with this "newbie" to publishing non-fiction.

To all of you, thank you, more than you will know.

Introduction

On 23rd July 1348, in the parish of San Biagio, Italy, the stifling heat only intensified the putrid smell of decay that had spread across the town. In a modest, tidy home that was not out of harm's way from disease, lived a woman named Ursollina. She shed the tears of a grieving widow as she came to terms with the fact that she needed to have her will drawn up to protect her children. Ursollina's husband, Carinus, a parchment maker, had drafted his own will about two weeks earlier. The devastation of the Black Plague was upon them, and neither husband nor wife would survive.

The Plague reached the shores of Italy in January 1348, and by the winter of that same year, it would wipe out a third of the country's population. Efforts to reduce the spread of this disease would prove fruitless. In Florence, the streets were cleared of garbage and refuse, and anyone believed to be sick was forbidden entry into the city. Many escaped to the countryside, where the death toll seemed to be lower.

This illness was so highly contagious that one could be dead in a few days or as little as a few hours. While the rich may have been able to afford a funeral, the poor would often leave their dead in the streets. Households were destroyed and crops abandoned in the wake of this dreadful disease.

In desperation, people, both rich and poor, began making out their wills as they feared the inevitable. One of these people was a woman named Ursollina of San Biagio. Left not only a widow but a mother, Ursollina did so wisely. Simple wills were more typical of skilled craftsmen, leaving the more elaborate wills to the wealthy. Both decrees were written for these individuals who were healthy in mind and intellect, but sick in body. How awful it must have been, in a time when the plague left a death toll of almost 60% in some regions, to know that you and your family would only add to the mortality rate.

The Black Death left in its wake, lands filled with turbulence and emptiness. Materials were scarce, and prices for goods skyrocketed.

Those who could not find work turned to crime, abandoned children were mistreated, and the morality of the people was suffering greatly.

It is hard to imagine, in a world now filled with the wonders of modern medicine, what it must have been like to live in such an uncertain time. We have been blessed over the past one thousand years with the continuing knowledge of physicians to understand and treat the human body. Man has learned how to stop bacteria in its tracks with the invention of antibiotics, and we've learned to replace the valve in one's heart with that of a pig or a cow. We now understand the importance of a sterile environment, and we've learned to treat psychiatric diseases that were once believed to be a form of possession.

In the time since William the Conqueror, through the reign of Henry VIII, significant advances have been made. In 1242, Muslim scholar, Ibn al Nafis, came to understand pulmonary and coronary circulation. In the late fifteenth century, Italian physician Antonio Benivieni, pioneered the use of autopsy. The Hippocratic oath states that a physician will *do no harm* and *abstain from intentional wrongdoing*. And while we may look at some practices of medieval medicine as atrocious, I do believe that physicians took that oath seriously.

Medicine, as well as history, particularly medieval, has always been a topic of utter fascination to me. I've long been intrigued by the spread of disease and the birthing process. I've continued to seek answers to why things were done the way they were in a time when electricity was centuries upon centuries away. I've continuously been fascinated by the history of treating the mentally ill.

After years of research, I've traced my own family's lineage through countless noblemen, back to the military commanders that served directly under Henry VII. And while my research has helped me to understand that my ancestors may have had better access to the latest medical breakthroughs of the time, most western Europeans did not have that luxury.

In writing this book, I've been given a chance to research in-depth the regimen for draining pustules and gain more knowledge of the exact role of the birthing chair. I've been able to take a fascinating journey down the road of bloodletting and to understand what was meant by an imbalance of the humours. I have been able to get more of a grasp of the unrelenting strength of the women who went through a truly natural childbirth. And I've also been able to build upon my fascination for the perils of the medieval battlefield.

In writing this book, I also look forward to enticing you, my reader, to expand your search in the knowledge of a topic that has been a favourite of mine since I can remember. I'll walk you through the origins of medicine dating back to Ancient Greek civilizations and explore some of the great minds behind medicine. I'll help you to understand the power the Catholic Church had on the sick and dying. Together we will grasp the importance of social structure and living conditions and better understand the role hierarchy had in preventing the spread of disease. You'll be able to understand just why the plague was so very deadly and why people did more to inhibit its growth than stop it. I hope to help women grasp some concept of the terrifying ordeal of childbirth, and I will elaborate on the rise of hospitals and the treatment of the mentally ill.

While historically, the Middle Ages are said to date from the fifth to the fifteenth century, you'll find that I often refer to happenings into the middle of the sixteenth century. I feel that the Renaissance made such advancements in medicine that it would be a disservice not to give credit to them. I've also been questioned as to why I chose to include torture and execution in a book on medieval medicine. The simple answer is because I wanted to. I was determined to find a connection between the two, if even to quench my thirst for stories on the macabre. But I genuinely believe there is a connection. The Middle Ages were a time of death and dying. While there was the business of keeping you alive through medicine, there was also a keen understanding that death was always around the corner. Folks in the Middle Ages understood the body much more than they were given credit for. They tried to understand what kept you alive, but also, they certainly understood ways to kill you. I feel there is such a secure connection between the two because one was either trying to avoid death or being forced to embrace it. People knew what hurt you, both emotionally and physically. So maybe torture and execution were used as a way to remind you that while your life was worth saving, it could also be taken from you in the blink of an eye.

I hope this book serves as a tool to engage my readers to share the passion I have always had in the history of medicine in the Middle Ages. I often stop and think if there was any way that I would have survived the times had I been born at the time of my ancestors.

Chapter One

A Foundation for Western Medicine is Built

I've always felt that to truly comprehend all that medicine has done for humans over the centuries, we need to stop and appreciate the great minds that built its foundation. These are the people whose genius provided the infrastructure that has kept us alive throughout time. While the history of the world is full of stories of great famine and the spread of disease, it is because of the continued knowledge of man that we continue to thrive.

Medicine and the human body remain a fascinating subject to this very day, and medical professionals continue to spin the wheel of knowledge in their desire to treat and cure disease. As humans, we have a desire to understand the mystery of our bodies and possess an internal propensity to make things right again when they fall out of order.

Since the beginning of time, I believe there has been an undomesticated need for all mammals to nurture. Whether through the mothering instincts of primates or the proven emotional awareness of elephants, creatures have always held within them a need for survival and protection of their most vulnerable.

The history of medicine dates to roughly 7000 BCE, when the Neanderthals are believed to have possibly practised some form of medicine. The remains of our archaic relatives reveal that they suffered some horrendous injuries. Calamities that probably arose from warfare or hunting accidents, or trying to escape the jaws of predators are visible on fossils. But despite the broken limbs and crushed skulls that fill the exhibits of natural history museums, these individuals managed to survive for quite some time after their injuries. History would have us assume that the Neanderthals were nothing but dense prehistoric beings who lacked the necessary intellect and cognitive skills. But if we look at the fact that they did somehow survive almost imminent death, we can examine the notion that they must have had some understanding of how to care for one another. There is supporting evidence that Neanderthals

2   Medicine in the Middle Ages

may have developed skills such as midwifery and wound dressing, as well as harnessing some understanding of the medicinal purposes of plants. There are records of medicine being practised in Mesopotamia during the Third Dynasty of Ur, beginning in the year 2112 BCE. These people were believed to have been aptly trained for their time, possessing the tools and pharmaceuticals to treat the sick. As early as 3100 BCE, the Ancient Egyptians developed medicine in both the study of the body and in diagnostics. The Egyptians understood the challenge of setting broken bones and administering dentistry as well as minimally invasive surgery. The Early Iron Age of India, beginning in 1500 BCE, provides some of the earliest texts of medicine, documented in *The Atharvaveda*, one of the first Hindu texts that contained various herbal remedies. Traditional Chinese medicine has been observed through Taoist physicians for at least twenty-three centuries, through the study of disease and illness.

However, it was the study of medicine in Greek, Roman, and Muslim countries that provides the basis for the understanding of the practice of medicine during the Middle Ages. This period in history is usually understood as the time between 500 BCE throughout the year 1500 BCE in Europe. Beginning with the fall of the Roman Empire, medieval history is categorised into the early, high, and late Middle Ages. The acceptance of medical knowledge into western civilization was conditioned by several social factors that spanned over time.

Life was hard for many people who lived in Ancient Greece, performing their day-to-day duties under the warmth of the dry climate. While many people made a living by farming and fishing, land and water could often be scarce. But cities in Greece also thrived with temples made of stone and beautiful theatres where people would gather. Greece was also the birthplace of several philosophers who used abundant logic and reason to study the world around them. These philosophers were mathematicians and scientists who laid the foundation for what many consider the essence of life. Among these intellectuals who contributed to Greek society were several practitioners of medicine.

Ancient Greek medicine was a collaboration of practices and theories that were constantly changing throughout time. While illness was believed to be a punishment from the divine, over time, there became a need to understand the material causes. Practitioners took a greater interest in understanding the body and illness itself as well as the connection between the cause of the affliction and the most effective treatments. They began to realize that health was affected by several contributing factors, including diet, society, geographic location, as well as one's own beliefs and personal traumas. And while practitioners came to understand the body, they still believed strongly in the role of the divine when it came to illness and the healing of disease. The Greek practitioners of medicine also believed strongly in the function of the humours. *The Theory of Humourism* conceived that the human body was made up of a balance of four humours: blood, phlegm, yellow and black bile. Practitioners believed that good health resulted from a perfect balance of these humours and that poor health resulted in an imbalance of them.

Myths in Ancient Greece espouse the first physician to be Asclepius, the son of Apollo, the god of healing and medicine. Asclepius's mother was believed to have been a mortal woman named Coronis. A common myth says that Coronis was killed for infidelity while pregnant with Apollo's son. Apollo, wanting to save his child, cut him from the womb. Asclepius learned many things not only from his father but from the mythological centaur, Chiron, who gave him much of his formal medical education. With his birth dating back before 350 BCE, Asclepius grew to be a gifted healer. He is said to have provided healing centres, specifically *The Temple of Asclepius*, that boasted springs that offered healing powers to those that drank or bathed in its water. Simple surgeries and the draining of abscesses have also taken place in these temples. Myths also say that Asclepius was so gifted a healer that he eventually overshadowed his father and his teacher. There are tales of Asclepius saving people on the brink of death with his power and his knowledge.

The Rod of Asclepius, a snake wrapped around a staff, is the universal symbol of medicine used today. The origin of the rod stems back to the vast healing temples of Asclepius, where a non-venomous snake was used to slither around the floors, surrounding the sick and dying. Asclepius brought these same snakes with him at the founding of each new temple. Countless stories of his healing spread, and people began to flock to his temples to be cured. The symbol of the snake and staff is now the official logo of the World Health Organization. But the Rod of Asclepius is not to be confused with Caduceus, a rod depicting two snakes and a pair of wings, while the Rod of Asclepius has only one snake and no wings.

4 Medicine in the Middle Ages

Surrounded by aqua-coloured water and boasting sandy white beaches lies the island of Kos, Greece, the birthplace of Hippocrates of Kos (460 BCE–375 BCE). Hippocrates was a Greek physician who lived during Greece's Classical period and is known as The Father of Medicine. Born to wealthy parents and a physician father, Hippocrates was likely given a proper education before continuing his studies in the field of medicine. Like Asclepius, he learned from his father. His medical training is also attributed to the Greek physician, Herodicus, who is associated with sports medicine. Historians believed that Hippocrates travelled throughout much of Greece practising medicine and perhaps into Egypt and Libya as well. Hippocrates lived in a time when most people felt that illness was tied to superstition and the wrath of the gods. But he discovered that disease had a root cause and went on to use this philosophy as the foundation of his teachings.

The Hippocratic Corpus is a collection of roughly sixty ancient Greek medical writings associated with Hippocrates and his teachings. These writings include the texts of not only Hippocrates but other physicians who practised at the same time he did. These medical texts supply us with some of the oldest examples of Greek writings. A unique aspect of these writings teaches the same underlying assumptions on how the body, as well as disease, worked. *The Hippocratic Corpus* contains scientific consideration of Hippocrates and his teaching through observation and treatment. The producers of writings based on Hippocrates were often very keen observers who would describe symptoms of disease along with the recommended course of treatment. These texts supported many different aspects of medicine, not only through the physician but the apothecary as well. It examined treatment from the view of the simple layperson, who was looked at more as someone who could speak with the doctor regarding the patient. Hippocratic medicine laid the groundwork for what we still know today to be accurate; that a proper diet and physical exercise can work wonders for the body and many of its ailments. Though it may have been elaborated on over time, it is Hippocrates who is genuinely credited with *The Theory of the Four Humours*.

Hippocrates believed that the four humours represented the four major liquids in the body: yellow bile, black bile, blood, and phlegm. He associated each humour with one of the four elements and believed that an imbalance of these humours would cause illness and distress in the body. Hippocrates taught that the interactions among the four humours, along with the weather and the placement of the planets, would ultimately determine not only a person's physical health but their mental status as well. He believed that a person's personality was also greatly affected by the balance or imbalance of the four humours.

Hippocrates attributed yellow bile to a choleric disposition as well as associating it with fire or the summer. He believed that yellow bile was related to hot and dry qualities and was directly attributed to the function of the gallbladder. Yellow bile was also associated with childhood. According to Hippocrates, black bile was related to a somewhat melancholic disposition and associated with the earth and winter. Black bile was cold and dry and had a relation to the spleen, as well as old age. Blood was related to a sanguine or overly social personality and linked to the qualities of hot and moist. It was believed to be connected to the air and to spring and possess the attributes of adolescence. Hippocrates taught that phlegm was part of a phlegmatic disposition, one where a person was relaxed and compassionate. Phlegm possessed the qualities of cold and moist and was linked to water, the brain, and one's maturity.

The Hippocratic Corpus contains a text of written work called *Sacred Disease*, which supports Hippocrates' argument that not all disease derived from supernatural sources. This theory was the fundamental source for his belief that good health came from a proper balance of the body's four humours. Being too hot or too cold or being dry or wet would much disturb the balance of the humours, resulting in sickness and disease. The definition of the very word disease is *imbalance*. Physicians who followed this theory believed that bringing the body into balance again was the right path to regaining one's health.

The Greek people had a philosophy of rational and natural medicine, which was made up of a radical approach to disease and healing. The authors of Hippocratic medicine often criticised traditional beliefs. Such conventional views were ideas that relied on theology and mythology. In the Greek period of cultural history, earthly and religious forms of healing succeeded quite well together.

The birthplace of Hippocrates had become the birthplace of medicine primarily in the fifth century. It was also the centre of worship for Asclepius. Asclepius is said to have appeared in the dreams of those that slept in the shrines of Kos. Through their dreams, physicians could obtain great medical advice directly from Asclepius that would guide them in their journey to treat the ill.

Aristotle (384 BCE–322 BCE), the ancient Greek philosopher and scientist, was equally important to the rise of medicine. Aristotle was born in Stagira, a small village off the southern part of Greece. Both Aristotle's parents came from traditional families, and because his parents passed away when he was young, he was likely raised by family at his home in Stagira. At age seventeen, Aristotle enrolled in the Academy of Plato. Plato (428 BCE–348 BCE), the Athenian philosopher, expanded on the ideas of his own teacher, Socrates (470 BCE–399 BCE). Aristotle would become Plato's most exceptional student and an equally crucial Greek philosopher.

Aristotle was known for insisting there was a relationship between natural philosophy and medicine. He had made countless observations of the world around him, precisely the day-to-day habits of plants and animals. Aristotle is credited with identifying over 500 species of animals. He deemed that all animals, from small plants to human beings, were arranged on a scale of perfection and believed that a creature's accomplishments were seen in its form and biology. He also divided biology into three separate types of souls: vegetative, sensitive, and rational. A vegetative soul was capable of growth, a sensitive soul was responsible for movement and sensation, and a rational soul was one of thought and consideration.

Aristotle was also the founder of *Lyceum*, an Athenian school of Peripatetics, in a grove sacred to Apollo. True to its name, Aristotle would walk about the orchard lecturing to his students. Through abundant discussion and his quest for scientific knowledge, Aristotle influenced much of the writings of medicine.

During his time teaching, Aristotle took Theophrastus, a Greek student, under his wing. Under his tutelage, Theophrastus (371 BCE–287 BCE) would become Aristotle's successor at the Lyceum. Theophrastus was incredibly knowledgeable about botany and would go on to write a series of books called *The History of Plants*. Many of his names for plants would survive well into modern times.

Aristotle's significant influences are present in the writings of Galen (129 CE–210 CE), a Greek physician, surgeon and philosopher, who thrived during the Roman Empire. The son of a wealthy architect, Galen was fortunate to receive an extensive education that would prepare him for his successful career as a philosopher and physician. Galen's understanding of medicine was based on the theory of humourism, much like the teachings of Hippocrates. Galen also took an interest in the opinions of the Greek physicians Herophilus (335 BCE–280 BCE) and Erasistratus (304 BCE–250 BCE). Both Herophilus and Erasistratus were known for their pioneering into the field of anatomy and dissection. They were responsible for opening a school of anatomy in Alexandria, where Herophilus became the first medical teacher. Herophilus was able to distinguish between veins and arteries and their role in the body. Herophilus and Erasistratus both became engaged in the dissection of the deceased and ultimately performed autopsies. They were also given criminals on which they were able to conduct examinations while they were still alive. They were able to identify the brain as well as the nervous system.

The Greek founders of medicine had several diverse approaches to the way they viewed medicine. These approaches consisted of the Rationalist, Empiricist, and Methodical belief systems. The system of Rationalism believed that the primary task of a physician was to investigate the cause of disease. It was based on an appropriation of knowledge through experience. The Empirical approach believed that the only task of doctors was to treat patients based on their experience. The Methodical approach to medicine was the belief that all medical treatment could be carried out in simple rules that could be learned in a short amount of time.

Greek Medicine reached its fullest developments through the teachings of Galen. He was one of the greatest minds in science to date and has remained unsurpassed. His writings brought together the heritage of Greek medicine. He also supported the teachings of Hippocrates in believing that the best doctor is also one who is a philosopher. Galen has been said to have credited the teachings of Hippocrates over that of Aristotle. Galen's anatomical work, which usually consisted of the study of monkeys and pigs, was the driving force behind his personal theories. Along with the work of his predecessors, Galen's opinion took the Rationalist approach, and he even argued against the doctrine of the Empiricist approach. He placed a tremendous amount of value on his subjective observations.

The origins of Greek medicine carried over to the Roman Empire, and much of the belief system of the Romans was very "Greek" in nature.

8 Medicine in the Middle Ages

Throughout the sixth century, schools in Alexandria were built and based on the teachings of Galen, as several Roman doctors had Greek origins.

Latin writers, such as Aulus Cornelius Celsus (25 BCE–50 CE), drew significantly upon Greek sources. Celsus is known for his expert work on diet, pharmaceuticals, and medical-related fields. Cities throughout the Roman Empire became supplied with doctors whose education was based predominantly on Greek society and teachings.

However, during the first three centuries of the Christian era, very few Greek teachings were translated into Latin. There simply wasn't a need for it. It wasn't until the later years before the Middle Ages that politics, along with culture, closed the gap between Western and Eastern parts of the world. In the west, there was becoming an interest in medicine for more practical purposes, which called for more translation. The full translation of Greek medical text truly began in the fifth century. And so, by the sixth century, there was becoming more Hippocratic and Galenic works translating into Latin. These conversions made it possible for readers to get a general understanding of the inner workings of Greek medicine. Greek medicine taught Romans the importance of diet and gave terminology to diseases. It also provided much information on treatments, as well as the female reproductive system. But the medical literature that was available during the early Middle Ages had only a few Greek sources.

By the end of the fourth century, Christianity was officially established as the religion of the Roman Empire. It was shaped by not only the belief in the supernatural but also on the idea that nature could be manipulated. The Roman Catholic Church played an enormous role in the western development of medicine. This gave promise to the belief in religious healing and the rise of monasteries. Monasteries provided a new look at the way medicine was viewed and learned. Christians believed that sickness was an evil in life, and medicine was considered a new birth in the fall of man. However, there did remain differing opinions on whether illnesses were genuinely attributed to the sins of man. Jesus Christ did not adhere to the thought process that disease was a direct result of sin.

Still, there have been Christian commentaries that have interpreted things as divine reckoning. Pope Gregory (540–604), who became Pope in the year 590 CE, and who was most known for converting the Pagan Anglo-Saxons in England to Christianity, believed that plagues were the result of the sin of man. Many early Christians felt that any illness received was the will of God and needed to be accepted. However, Christians also believed that disease was a result of natural environmental factors.

Christianity was a religion that strongly believed in divine intervention and healing. The care of sick individuals was viewed as a charity, and one was thought to be doing the work of God through their own hands. While the study of medicine was encouraged in Christianity, it was also about caring for humanity. It was assumed that in addition to spiritual healing, the role of the monk was to tend to the sick and dying. True to the foundation of Christianity, the Benedictine Monk St. Augustine (early sixth century) preached that Jesus Christ was the true healer and physician.

Though not as widely documented, the role of the Jewish practitioner did carry significant influence throughout the Middle Ages. Many of the advances made respecting women and childbirth during the Middle Ages can be attributed to Jewish text. Although many of these texts were written in the masculine form of Hebrew and believed to be directed at male physicians, female practitioners made significant contributions to communities, both Jewish and non-Jewish. Judging from these texts, it appears that the most significant contribution made by Jewish women was during the fourteenth and fifteenth centuries. And yet still, despite this, substantial limitations were inflicted upon them by society. Christian Universities refused both Jewish men and women. And so, the education of women especially fell on the shoulders of others. Because Jewish doctors were educated in Greek, Arabic, or Hebrew, this gave them the advantage of acquiring and understanding medical texts that were out of reach from their Christian peers. Jewish women were exceptionally skilled in midwifery and made up a more significant percentage in some regions. During the period between 1390–1415, there were twenty-four Jewish midwives in the French town of Marseille, as opposed to only eighteen Christian midwives. But the degree to which Jewish women practised midwifery largely depended on the region they were from. Despite their contribution to medicine, Jewish women still faced discrimination due to not only their religion but their gender as well.

As the population increased over time, the needs of the cities grew enough so that Western monks began to seek out the chance to advance their medical knowledge and sharpen their skills. One of the most important developments in medicine during the seventh and eleventh centuries took place in the thriving Muslim communities throughout the Middle East. For six centuries, the writings of both St. Augustine and Hippocrates taught Christians to be faithful only to God's power and mystery. As far as Christians were concerned, there was no other reason to explore anything else, as they held firm to the belief that God was the only driving force in their lives. But as medical literature was translated into Arabic from Greek, Arabic doctors learned to absorb this material and build upon it. In stark contrast to the European way of life, Muslims have always put great importance on cleanliness. During the First Crusade to the Holy Land in 1096, as the Western army reached the East, Arabs were sickened by the stench of the Christian soldiers and their disregard for personal hygiene.

As higher education became increasingly structured during the ninth century, many major Muslim cities began to possess more and more universities. Students were taught the importance of cleanliness to stop the spread of disease, and they were instructed about the setting of bones and treating cataracts. They learned how to dispense medication. Muslim doctors followed the Hippocratic Oath and stressed that a true physician must be pious and disciplined. The development and advancement of hospitals were also of utmost importance to Muslim society.

Avicenna (980–1037), known to Muslims as Ibn Sina, was considered one of the most significant philosophers and thinkers during The Islamic Golden Age. One of his monumental contributions was his text *Canon of Medicine*. This text possessed a series of sections; general medicine, an overview of medications, diagnosing and treating of disease locally as well as conditions that spread through the body. It was throughout Avicenna's writings that Arabic medicine began to move west. The *Canon of Medicine* was later translated into Latin and today remains a central resource for medicine.

Although both Europe and the Muslim world received much of their knowledge from Greek sources, it was used differently. Arabic scholars had more access to much of the Greek texts, including Galen. However, Islamic medicine combined Galen's humourism with the practices of Persians, Hindus, and Arabs. This combination helped fulfil their need also to heal and comfort the sick. A large part of the intellect of Arab doctors was their receptiveness to new ideas, something the west struggled to accept. Islam's emphasis on the cleanliness of its people and society proved noteworthy advances in the health system. Muslim doctors were extremely skilled observers who relied much on the human body itself as opposed to archaic texts. They were pioneers in the diagnosing of disease and pharmacology. Avicenna's ground-breaking understanding of medicine, along with the pioneers in Islamic medicine, helped to get the west where it is today. Western medicine owes much to the Muslim world, and yet it took European physicians far too long before it was gratefully recognised.

Medicine in Greek origin looked at the body as a whole and strived to embrace all its workings. The Greeks believed that humans were essentially a part of what made up the universe, and they thought that planetary influences were part of what made up our health. While they were weary of the pagan overtones of such a thought process, early Christians also accepted this idea. But they were very cautious about practising anything that questioned the will and power of God. Beginning in the 1200s, more text became available from Greek, Hebrew, and Arab scholars that was morally questionable. But throughout the growth and development of scholars in the field of medicine, these ideas became more readily accepted.

By the fifteenth century, there became more and more text stressing the importance between human beings and the cosmos. Studies of astrology were translated from Arabic to Latin, beginning in the twelfth century. European doctors merged the teachings of Galen with the study of the stars. At the end of the 1500s, physicians were required to refer to the position of the moon before carrying out any complicated medical procedure. Many doctors were also becoming trained astrologers and used astrology in the diagnosis and treatment of their patients. They soon looked at one's horoscope as a part of the diagnosis. They contemplated the sequence of the planets from the time a patient was born, as well as their placement during the time of the illness. The astrology chart done for King Henry VIII (1491–1547) was relatively accurate. It said that Henry would be a cheerful, flirty child but the chart also warned of excessive personality traits. The chart predicted his short temper, sensitivity to criticism, his appetite for food, as well as his appetite for lust. Dr Lewis Caerleon (1465–1495) was a doctor and astronomer to Lady Margaret Beaufort (1441–1509), as well as her son, Henry VII (1457–1509), and his wife Queen Elizabeth of York (1466–1503). He was highly valued for his skills and was the recipient of generous favours from the Church.

Astrologers believed that the movement of the stars influenced things on earth, like the weather and the growth of crops. Almost all doctors had learned *The Doctrine of the Twelve Signs*, a text that described the relationship between the twelve zodiac signs and specific organs or limbs of the human body. *Zodiac Man* was a fifteenth century diagram of the human body that represented a correlation of the zodiacal names with certain body parts. It was used in texts on astrology, as well as calendars and the devotional *Book of Hours*. Doctors used the diagram in the fifteenth century as a means to determine the best time for bloodletting, surgery, and other procedures used to treat a patient. It was believed that when the cosmos were aligned with certain astrological signs that it drew a link to a bodily system or the four humours. It was only through a profound understanding of the cosmos that a doctor could decide whether their treatment would be lifesaving. By the 1500s, one could expect that an average physician would possess at least some understanding of the cosmos. Still, it was a select group of professionals that grasped an in-depth knowledge of astrology and how it affected medicine. With reference to the zodiac signs, the groundwork was laid for a great excuse if a patient didn't survive. A physician simply claimed that it was out of their hands, as the stars predetermined everything.

From the year 1050, not long before the Norman Conquest, the development of European society began to increase rapidly. The rise in expansion was a result of the increasing population and the growth of economics, as well as the building of schools. All these things played a vital part in how medicine was studied. The circulation of goods had advanced, and through translation into Latin, interest in the medical profession grew. So much of the new distribution of books was intellectually stimulating and sophisticated. As the twelfth century advanced, even more information became available. As Europeans began to accept the importance of astrology, there was slowly becoming a solid foundation on which to practice medicine. As populations grew, so did the spread of disease throughout the thirteenth and fourteenth centuries, giving scholars and physicians even more to ponder as they navigated the waters of medicine. And with the Renaissance spreading rapidly, it seemed as though Europe was dawning on a new and exciting medical era.

Chapter Two

The Influence of Christianity Spreads

The expansion of Christianity played an essential role as it began to dominate all aspects of life throughout medieval Europe. The founders of Christianity were adamant in their desire to spread the word of Jesus Christ, and they did so, not only through spoken word and text but also through their establishment of monasteries and hospitals.

Beginning in the Middle East with the very first followers of Jesus Christ, Christianity started its advancement along the shores of the Mediterranean and into other parts of the Roman Empire. Around the year 250 CE, the Romans were beginning their prosecution of early Christians. The idea of Christ as the new sovereign clashed with the notion that the Romans already had a sovereign, Julius Caesar (100 BCE–44 BCE). The fierce Roman dictator and military general was believed by many to have been lifted to heaven at his time of death and sent to live with the gods. The Roman people demanded loyalty to the state and viewed their emperor as their god. When Christians began to move their activities to more quiet locations such as their homes or shops, the Romans saw this as a privatisation of religion. It also gave the Romans a reason to prosecute them. But by the beginning of the fourth century, the prosecution of the Christians was coming to an end in The Roman Empire.

Constantine the Great (272 CE- 337 CE), who ruled between 306 CE and 312 CE, became the first Roman Emperor to convert to Christianity. It was under his rule that Christianity became the official religion of the Roman Empire. In the early centuries of this new religion, the bishops of Rome declared themselves the head of the Church. These Roman bishops, known as Popes, had a considerable influence over life in the early Middle Ages. However, they were still under the control of the mighty Byzantium Empire. Roman Popes felt it was their duty to convert the rest of Western Europe to Christianity.

The Roman churches eventually did break off from the Eastern Mediterranean sect, and the new church became known as the Roman

14 Medicine in the Middle Ages

Catholic and Roman Orthodox Church. Word of this church quickly spread through Ireland, and by the year 400 CE, there was a strong Christian presence in the country. Saint Patrick is said to have led great efforts to convert most of the population in the fifth century. Steadily, Christian communities were forming, and this prompted Ireland to spread the faith throughout the continent of Europe.

It was during the seventh century that the Irish, as well as the Roman Papacy, began to convert parts of Anglo Saxon England to Christianity. However, parts of England still reverted to Paganism as the Vikings started their invasion during the ninth and tenth centuries.

Clovis I (466 CE-511 CE), who was the ruler of the Germanic-speaking people, the Franks, was one of the first converts to Christianity. The land of the Franks is known today as France, Belgium, and Western Germany. Clovis was born a pagan but converted to Christianity in the year 496. His conversion was a significant milestone in establishing Christianity throughout Europe. It was during the ninth century, after pressure from the Carolingian Empire to convert, that most of the Saxons eventually did begin to follow Christ. Missionaries attempted to bring the religion to parts of Scandinavia during the ninth century, but they didn't truly accept it until after the early Middle Ages. As missionaries moved on through Iceland in the tenth century, it was a struggle to convince all the people to convert from the Norse faith. Although Christianity did eventually become official, the Norse faith could still be practised without fear of persecution. During the ninth and tenth centuries, Bulgaria loosely converted as well as Mieszko (930 CE-992 CE), the ruler of Poland, bringing Christianity to his nation. The Byzantines were making an effort to continue their movement through other parts of Europe, including Ukraine and Russia, in the ninth century. It was in 986 CE that Vladimir the Great (958 CE-1015 CE) began to follow the Church. Around this time, King Stephan (975 CE-1038 CE) of Hungary launched the promotion of Christianity and began to punish those who didn't follow through. It was throughout the twelfth and fourteenth centuries that Lithuania became one of the last countries to convert.

By 1054, one of the only universal institutions in Europe was the Church. While England was becoming a Christian country since Roman times, the Normans had also been Christian for a long time. In 1066, after the Battle of Hastings, William of Normandy (1028–1087) conquered England. He believed that it was important for the churches to come under Norman control. William was a devout Christian who went to great lengths to spread Christianity throughout England. While he accepted the Archbishop of Canterbury as the leader of the Church, William was also determined that it should be under his control. Along with William, most of the Normans who arrived with him in England were also devout Christians.

Christianity became the dominating force when it came to religion in the Middle Ages. The attempts to spread the faith throughout Europe had proved successful, but it was the Catholic Church, especially that soon became the only church. The Catholic Church played a role in the building of cathedrals and universities. It also became the law of the land, as Church leaders were also prominent roles in government. The powers of the Pope rose above all else, even higher than the monarchs. The lives of people during the Middle Ages became utterly dominated by the Catholic Church. With this knowledge, leaders of the Church made several attempts at turning its people against any other religion that crossed its path. The goal of Church leaders and their warriors was to make the world free of anyone who wasn't a Christian. While the Church had a history of denouncing Paganism, the Jews became the greatest threat to Christianity. Hatred was quickly spread by insisting that the Jews were responsible for the crucifixion of Christ, and many European countries issued a complete ban on them. Islam was also perceived as a threat to Christianity. Islamic ideas and innovation contributed immensely to the world through architecture and science, but in 1095, Pope Urban II (1035–1099) declared a holy war on Islam. The Church had used its own people as scapegoats by assuring them that by joining the holy war, they would be forgiven for their sins. In a world monopolised by religion and the fear of being labelled a heretic, thousands united in the fight against other religions.

Because Christians faced their own persecution during the Roman Empire and were forced to practice their faith in private, remote communities began to form in the fourth century. These were groups of people who believed in living a life of prayer and devotion and turning away from all worldly goods. Members of these communities initially lived together in a type of building constructed for hermits, where they committed to a life of solidarity and gathered for religious services. An *abba*, or abbot, presided over these individuals. They were eventually given the name *monachos*, derived from the Greek word *mono*, meaning one. The term mono is the origin of the word monk, which these people were eventually called.

Although there were monasteries that began to form in Egypt as early as the third century, it was throughout the fifth century that the idea of monasteries began to spread through Western Europe. These teachings were based on the Italian saint Benedict of Nursia (480–547). Saint Benedict was a monk himself and the founder of the monastery at Monte Cassino in Italy. He established a series of rules that encouraged members of his monastery to live as pure a life as possible. This regulation became known as the Benedictine order and instructed that monks live with only basic food and accommodations and very few personal possessions. Monks were responsible for the physical labour that would make the monastery self-sufficient. As these monasteries grew over time, donations from the wealthy would allow the monks to focus more on their scholarly duties, such as producing documents, and less time was given to general labour.

The daily lives of monks varied somewhat in accordance with the size of the monastery. Some housed around a dozen or so, while others could boast almost 500 men. An abbot was selected to lead his peers. He was often accompanied by a prior, who would assist in the administrative duties of the organization. Monks lived reasonably simple lives and were usually not permitted to leave the grounds of the monastery. From dusk until dawn, their lives were dictated by religious service. They wore modest clothing and were taught to forgo items of personal property. The number of monks living in the monastery would change their need for specific building structures, but most designs were entirely consistent. The monastery centred around the cloister, an area where inhabitants could talk amongst themselves and perform basic chores. These buildings usually had vast storage areas for food and wine, as well as a refectory where monks would take their meals. There were stables and general meeting rooms along with libraries. The structure was similar to a large manor house that tended to the needs of its own as well as others.

As monasteries began to acquire more wealth through increased taxes and donations, their power began to grow as well. Monasteries provided the locals with not only spiritual guidance but safety. Monasteries could give alms to the poor as well as looking after orphans and the sick. The

Benedictine monks followed a strict code that stated that they would care for the sick above and before every other duty. Monasteries usually had a separate infirmary along with impressive gardens filled with herbs that would aid in their care for the unwell.

During the Middle Ages, the Catholic Church dominated almost all aspects of life. Any different view was said to be heresy, and one could be punished for it. The Church also believed that any illness one might encounter was a direct punishment from God. If you fell ill, it was because of your sins. As the indoctrination of the Church continued to spread, people became fanatical about the idea of getting into God's Kingdom. One's deep belief in God would significantly affect decisions made regarding their health and treatment from their physicians. Medieval Christendom was initially divided into two parts; Eastern European Christianity under Constantinople and Western European Christianity, which fell under the rule of the Pope. When the Western Church banned marriage among all clerics, there was a considerable disagreement between the two sects, and in 1054, it caused them to split entirely. The Catholic Church controlled vast amounts of wealth during the Middle Ages as well as being the most prominent landowner. The Church expected a tithing, 10% of all income, to go directly to it. The Church monopolised education as well as acting as advisors to monarchs.

One of the most famous examples of the Church's power over its monarchs is that of Thomas Wolsey (1473–1530). Born March 1473 in Suffolk, Wolsey was the son of a butcher. In March 1498, he became an ordained priest after attending Magdalen College. He was introduced to King Henry VII in 1507 and became his appointed chaplain. When Henry VIII ascended to the throne after the death of his father, Wolsey was appointed his Royal Almoner. The young king took great favour with Wolsey and began to entrust more power to him, and followed his counsel on matters of the state. While Henry spent his early time as king embracing his love for sportsmanship and hunting, Wolsey became his go-to man and was slowly becoming the power behind the throne. Henry continued to grant him great favours and proclaimed him Dean of York in 1513. The Pope appointed him Cardinal in 1515, and he was also named Lord Chancellor by the king. Aside from having the highest secular position, he now basked in an elevated position of the Church. In 1518, Wolsey was successful in forming an alliance between England, the Holy Roman Emperor, Charles V (1500–1558), Maximilian I (1459–1519), and Francis I of France (1494–1547). Wolsey was given the title *legatus a latere* by the Pope and became the most influential church official in England. His revenue would increase even more in 1518 when he was appointed Bishop of Bath and Wells. In what was one of the most extravagant creations in history, Wolsey arranged the Field of Cloth of Gold, where King Henry would meet the King of France.

The two young monarchs were still on edge with each other, despite their recent alliance. In an effort to outshine each other, no expense was spared on either side in their displays of wealth. Beautiful pavilions made of real cloth of gold had been constructed, along with jousting and other competitions. Lavish banquets were held, all in a means to impress one another. The splendour of festivities continued for three weeks. But despite his acquired wealth and rise to the top, Wolsey would fail to hold the king's favour forever. When his attempts at getting the king a divorce from his first wife continued to fall through, Henry would eventually abandon him by pulling most of his ranks and holding him prisoner. Wolsey died of natural causes before he could face further punishment from the king.

The Book of Hours, developed in the twelfth century, was a sacred prayer book that was popular during the Middle Ages. Whether it was used as a direct form of publicity from the Church is unknown, but if anything, it only secured the notion that people relied heavily on their faith. The origin of *The Book of Hours* stems from psalms that were recited by monks and nuns. It was a collection of beautifully enlightened illustrations, texts, prayers, and psalms. It was developed for the layperson who wished to touch upon the monastic life and incorporate it into their own. Some of these books contained images referencing the very people who carried it, along with the coats of arms of the said family. Each book was uniquely tailored to the individual, though they all included the *Hours of the Virgin Mary*. This was important as many of the books were made for women especially. They could be given as a wedding gift from a husband to his new bride or carried by a laywoman who had yet to marry. The goal of the book was to help one with spiritual life. This was in accordance with the eight canonical hours observed by all devout members of the Church. While most monarchs throughout the Middle Ages most likely possessed a *Book of Hours*, there are particular members of royalty who stand out as particularly pious. Lady Margaret Beaufort, mother to Henry VII, was well known for her reverence. One of her most special personal belongings was her own *Book of Hours*, known as *The Beaufort Book of Hours*. Her book contained a calendar of saints where she chose to record notable events in her own family, including the birth of her grandsons, Arthur and Henry Tudor. Perhaps one of the most admired *Book of Hours* is the one that belonged to Anne Boleyn (1501–1536). During her youth, Anne was the epitome of virtue and devotion, and her own personal *Book of Hours* proves just that.

There remain three copies of her prayer book, two of which are on display at Hever Castle, her childhood home. Anne's *Book of Hours* is of a higher quality than those owned by middle-class women. It is thought that she may have acquired one of them while she served the French Court as a teenager. Like Margaret Beaufort, Anne had written personal notes in the margins, either in French or in English. "Remember me when you do pray. That hope doth lead from day to day". This inscription was written alongside an illustration of the Virgin Mary, almost as a sign of Anne's innocence.

The Catholic Church understood its power as a propaganda machine and used it to great advantage. Demonic possession had always plagued humans throughout history, and the Church used it as controlling leverage in furthering its authority over the people of Western Europe. The Church had a firm understanding of the ignorance of people when it came to religion. This ignorance was a perfect opportunity for the Church to push the threat of possession. It also gave them the means to stress the need for exorcism. Possession was considered to be one of the most prominent reasons behind mental instability. The Church was a firm believer that demons were the driving force behind mania and epilepsy, which of course, was not understood but seen as another manifestation of demonic possession. Medieval medical texts write of an incubus who is a lustful demon who strangles its victims.

Along with the belief in demonic possession, there was also a physiological explanation. It was explained as an overabundance of black bile and a disease of the head as well as mania. Theologians also believed that evil spirits could cause melancholy, which fell in line with a physician's theory that evil spirits could cause an imbalance of the humours. What was believed to be the tell-tale signs of possession closely resembled the symptoms of physical unrest. Hysteria, or what was called uterine suffocation, echoed possession because of the mental confusion, grinding of teeth, and convulsions. Physicians believed that a woman's womb could become displaced, causing it to move about her body. They attributed this to witchcraft or demonic possession. Uterine suffocation, or wandering womb, was most likely nothing more than the result of a severe mental illness that wasn't understood. Epileptic fits would cause an individual to flail about and grind their teeth as well, leaving physicians and clerics to believe an evil spirit inhabited the patient.

The Church, as well as physicians, had their list of signs that would be typical for a diagnosis of possession. Abnormal convulsions, blasphemy regarding the saints or God, using religious symbols in an unhealthy way, and aggression not only towards themselves but others were common signs. The theory that one was possessed truly tested the boundaries between health and religion. In the Middle Ages, the thought that someone was dominated by an entity was sincerely terrifying, especially for those who were deeply religious. And although in several cases, an illness could be explained by medicine, the Catholic Church would often overshadow this notion. It was partly due to their attempt to gain greater control over the social and economic aspects of the lives of its patrons. Catholic authorities preached consistently that one's immortal soul was in jeopardy at all times, especially when trying to resist the temptations of the devil. The Church believed that any unexplainable or irrational event must be caused by an external force trying to make its way into the body. They deemed any deviant behaviour a result of possession. The threat of demonic possession only led to a higher authority for the Church. This constant reminder that your soul was vulnerable was the Church's way of having total control over the everyday social dynamics of not only small villages but most of Western Europe.

So many physicians blamed mental illness on possession, and so in most cases, the treatment was often left up to the clerics. Along with the use of scourging to cause physical pain, the Church often encouraged self-mutilation as a treatment. But if they believed that someone was indeed possessed, they would call for an exorcist. *Vade Retro Satana* was a formula that was written on performing an exorcism in 1415 by Benedictine monks in Bavaria. Early text mentions that even just making the sign of the cross over an individual would be enough for an exorcism.

Some narratives speak of prayers being said over the victim, along with the use of the Book of Psalms to help expel the devil. These narratives also mention that when confronted by an exorcising priest, this would cause the demon to become agitated, and the person may engage in violent behaviour. It is recorded that it was common for the victim to engage not only in physical altercations but to scream and shout obscenities.

Because the Middle Ages focused around the Church, one of the main things the family of the possessed might turn to was the healing works of a saint. The medieval saint was believed to have the ability to perform miracles, and exorcising a demon was one of those miracles. Exorcising a demon was looked at as a struggle against Satan. Some of the earliest stories in the Gospel refer to the exorcising of an evil spirit. Twelfth and thirteenth century texts are full of tales of demonic possession, and towards the second half of the twelfth century, these descriptions became quite expressive. Saints typically used three common defence mechanisms in the fight against evil: the cross, prayer along with the laying on of hands, and holy water. If expelling the demon became physical, then it was a blow intended for the beast and not the possessed person. When holy water was utilised, it could be sprinkled on the victim, but at times, they might be completely submerged. Often much time was devoted to the ritual as it was strenuous and time-consuming. It was entirely possible for a victim to be plagued by more than one entity at a time. These cases were long and complicated, and while one demon left the body, another could take its place. Several documented evidence of an exorcism that appears in hagiographic texts states that they took place after the death of the saint. Especially in the Middle Ages, the body of one who was possessed would be brought to the shrine of the chosen saint and left there. However, this could often be a deterrent to church visitors if screaming and gnashing of teeth took place during a sermon. But the ultimate wish was for a miracle, nonetheless. Medieval text describes, in many cases, a complete recovery of the possessed.

Often the victim recalled visions of the beloved saint, who exorcised the demonic one from their body. The victim wakes up from his or her reverie type sleep and finds they are pure once again. Several notable saints were said to cast out Satan from the possessed. Blessed William of Toulouse (1297–1369) was a noteworthy exorcist in France. St Benedict of Nursia cast out the devil with the sign of the cross. Saint Vincent

Ferrer (1350–1419) was a Dominican saint who, during his life, was the source of many extraordinary miracles, including delivering over seventy people from possession. Witnesses also claim that he raised almost thirty people from the dead. The sick and the dying flocked to Ferrer in hopes of a divine miracle.

In the Middle Ages, the ritual of exorcism was a part of what seemed like everyday life. During the twelfth century, there was a rise in the number of exorcisms performed. The purpose of a saint's life was seen as a means to fight the demon and grant people the gift of purification. While the first official guidelines for exorcism weren't established until 1614, when it was discovered that the ritual was being performed without the authority of the Church, the practice was undoubtedly a sought-after cure for a demonic soul. It wasn't until after the seventeenth century that intellectuals, as well as some church leaders, began to argue that such an experience was caused by psychology and science.

During the Middle Ages, with the Church's influence, deeming someone possessed was the perfect explanation for the enigmas of mental illness and neurological disorders that were not yet understood. It has become clear to us today how during a time when people relied almost solely on their faith, it was easy for the Church to have complete control over all walks of life. Folks who had little knowledge of the world outside their villages were dependent on God and on the prayers of the Church to keep them healthy. The spread of Christianity throughout medieval Europe thoroughly left its mark on the innocence of the people.

Chapter Three

A Hierarchy of Importance

If ever there was a time when family mattered, it was the Middle Ages. In a period filled with the turbulence of war and the constant threat of famine and disease, the ranking of your family mattered a great deal. It determined the manner in which you would spend your days, as well as the level of care you might receive if you became ill. If you were lucky enough to be born into great wealth, you could rest assured that you would most likely be spared the laborious hours spent working in the fields or clearing the streets of waste. But even if you weren't born into poverty, it didn't mean that your life would be safe from danger or disease. With a life expectancy of just over thirty-one years of age for a male, the world was full of imminent injury and illness no matter who you were. But you could at least have comfort knowing that if you were at the upper crust of society, you could afford the best medicine had to offer. People knew where they stood on the ladder of hierarchy, and everyone expected things to go accordingly.

Society as a whole during the Middle Ages was built on a system called feudalism. Most popular between the ninth and fifteenth centuries, feudalism was how society was structured around the holding of lands in exchange for services. Feudalism was a medieval way of life in which the lower class showed respect to the upper class. At the top of the social ladder always sat the monarch who had the ultimate decision on all things. Kings and queens were believed to be anointed by God and associated with the saints. They were often looked at as not only a protector of their people but as a healer as well. Wealthy, privileged nobles sat just under the king or queen.

Nobles were wealthy landowners who usually inherited their land. Nobles were influential in government and their homes and had control over those that worked for them. The knight was someone who was valued for their military valour. They were skilled warriors who were a constant presence at the homes of monarchs and nobles. Knights were different from average soldiers. They were better trained and usually came from a wealthy family. Because knights protected nobles, they were often rewarded with lands and manor houses of their own. Often thought of as middle class, merchants and skilled craftsmen played an essential role in society as well. Merchants often travelled to far lands to buy foreign goods to be sold at marketplaces. Marketplaces essentially became medieval towns beginning in the fourteenth century when merchants began storing their products in warehouses and hiring various kinds of skilled craftsmen to help turn their goods into profit. Serfs and peasants fell at the bottom of feudal society. Serfs especially owned no land and were forbidden to leave the manor they worked on without permission from their employer. In exchange for their hard labour, which usually consisted of working the fields, they were rewarded with a place to live, food, and protection from the landowner.

During the Middle Ages, there were fewer people just about everywhere. Almost 90% of people lived in villages that were scattered throughout the country connected by small roads or paths. Most people didn't travel beyond where they were born as they not only didn't have the money, but times were perilous. People feared attacks from robbers and thieves and felt safer surrounded by their villages. Much of a person's safety, whether from intruders or disease, depended on their social ranking. The lives of monarchs and nobles didn't differ too much when it came to their living accommodations. But the lives of the peasants were at the other end of the spectrum regarding not only safety but personal comfort and hygiene.

Kings, queens, and nobles were served with the most that luxury and safety had to offer. A majority of that safety was inside the walls of a castle. While the castle underwent drastic changes with respect to comfort since the eleventh century, it has always remained the safest place to live. And it has also remained the iconic picture of the living quarters of the wealthy during medieval times. Around the time of the Norman invasion, when some of the first castles were being built, they were simple wooden forts with a single tower. It wasn't until closer to the year 1100 that stone construction began. Castles would continue to improve significantly over the next 300 years; they would become larger, more comfortable, and better defended. Castles were constructed with an outer wall or a curtain wall that would enclose the entire structure. Often these walls were surrounded by large moats. Massive towers were built so any incoming invaders could be seen attacking the curtain wall. Some of these curtain walls were over twenty feet thick. The gatehouse of a castle was the most heavily defended area with heavy, steel doors. It possessed several openings for soldiers to shoot arrows at intruders, or worse, pour boiling water over them. The middle part of the castle was known as the keep, also heavily defended by soldiers. The keep was where the king, or noble, lived with his family and was the safest part of the castle. Castles also provided a safe haven for villagers in times of danger and offered protection for the servants and soldiers that served their lords.

While the wealthy and powerful certainly lived better than most, it still wasn't luxurious when held to today's standards, and an incredible amount of effort was put into keeping a castle clean and comfortable. That wasn't an easy feat. By design, castles were notoriously cold and damp. Of course, as we know today, a cold and wet environment is detrimental to one's health. Mould thrives in dank and poorly ventilated buildings where there is little to no heating and insulation. The cold, wet castle walls provided a perfect atmosphere for mould to accumulate. Inhaling mould spores inflamed the airway, causing congestion, wheezing, coughing, and throat irritation. Infants and the elderly were especially subject to sickness from these surroundings. The prolonged exposure to these conditions most likely caused asthma in more vulnerable people.

Because insulation was hundreds of years away, rushes were used to offer some barrier between one's feet and the cold stone floors. Rushes were a collection of dried plant stems and how they were used is the subject of some debate. Some historians will argue that they were simply tossed about the floor, while some suggest that the dried stems were woven together to form some sort of a mat. What we do know is that sweet-smelling herbs, such as lavender, were placed over the rushes so the scent would be released when being stepped on. However, rushes were also an excellent place to collect debris such as table scraps, spilt beer, grease, saliva, and dog and cat faeces. Rushes were also a perfect environment for rats and lice, as well as fleas. While rushes were replaced, it was usually just the top layer that was changed, and the bottom layer was left to fester. This trend may have proved more so in homes of lesser wealth, but one can imagine that castles were still subject to such breeding grounds of bacteria. As the Dutch Philosopher Erasmus (1466–1536) noted:

The floors are, in general, laid with white clay and are covered with rushes occasionally renewed, but so imperfectly that the bottom layer is left undisturbed, sometimes for twenty years, harbouring expectoration, vomit, the leakage of dogs and men, ale, droppings, scraps of fish and other abominations, not fit to be mentioned.

Fireplaces offered warmth, but they also offered a roomful of smoke, as not all had been designed for the smoke to rise up and out. So often, a warm room meant a smoky room. Long term exposure to smoke, as we know today, is deadly. What people didn't understand was that they were subjecting themselves to chronic cardiovascular diseases, heart attack, heart arrhythmia, asthma, and an almost certain premature death. Carbon monoxide, as well as benzene, formaldehyde, acrolein, and polycyclic aromatic hydrocarbons, make up only a few of the deadly chemicals that linger in smoke from burning wood.

Along with harmful toxins from particle pollution, is soot. Soot attacks the lungs and respiratory system, causing irritability. It gets into one's eyes and nose, damaging the sinuses. As with most undesirable living conditions, pregnant women and children were most vulnerable due to their developing respiratory systems.

Castles boasted few windows, which didn't let in a lot of sunlight, but also kept out some of the cold. Another effort to combat damp conditions was to hang tapestries on the castle walls or over the windows to keep out the cold. The wealthy also wore several layers of clothing to stay warm, even in the summer, and slept in elaborate beds covered with silk and velvet blankets

Royalty may have been treated with all the comforts available to them, but one thing they probably didn't have was running water. In 1236 in London, a 2.7-mile-long underground pipe was constructed that ran from Tyburn to Cheapside. This piping system carried water to a public fountain. There is also evidence that some monasteries and palaces may have had water tapped in, but as far as castles, it is doubtful. Naturally, no running water meant a very primitive toilet. Usually called a privy or garderobe, the medieval bathroom probably had minimal effort invested into it concerning privacy and waste disposal. Castle toilets were typically small and never any more prominent than they had to be. They were usually built into walls and projected out onto corbels. Any waste would fall below and into a castle's moat or its cesspit.

In some cases, the waste went directly into the river. The king and queen or lord of the castle were usually given the luxury of a private toilet, which was set back in a chamber or passage with a wooden door, but most everyone else had a chamber pot. The seat of the toilet consisted of a wooden bench that covered the shaft hole in the stone. Grass, hay, or moss was typically used as toilet paper. Some bathrooms may have offered a small window for fresh air, and the floor was most likely covered with rushes to provide some warmth. Walls were often whitewashed with lime plaster because it was understood that lime killed off bacteria. Like the rushes spread about the floors of the castle, they most likely provided a home for vermin, bacteria, and faecal matter to accumulate.

If you were lucky enough to live during Tudor times, you could have been awarded the highest position available in the king's Privy Chamber, Groom of the Stool. The role was created around 1495 by Henry VII, which was primarily tending to the king's personal needs. But it was his son, Henry VIII, who took it a step further. It was the job of the Groom of the Stool to monitor the king's bowel movements and report them to doctors. While it seems disgusting to us today, it was vital that the king's health was closely monitored. There is some dispute among historians, but it is believed that towards the end of his reign, Henry VIII had gotten so obese that the Groom of the Stool was instructed to wipe his bottom after his bowel movements.

Because almost no one, unless you were very wealthy, could afford a private bathtub, it was an absolute luxury to have one. Monarchs and nobles knew that luxury. Private baths were constructed of wooden tubs, where tent-like sheets hung over the top with flowers and sweet-smelling herbs like sage, marjoram, rosemary, and orange peel. Sponges or soft cushions were provided for the lord or lady to lay back on, and attendants would bring jugs of hot water. The tubs were filled with warm, fresh herbs used to wash, and if the master of the castle had aches, herbs like chamomile, brewer's wort, mallow, and fennel were boiled and added to the bath in the hopes of offering some relief.

There was much misconception over the importance of hygiene when it came to those at the top of the feudal system. King John of England (1199–1216) had his own personal bathtub and attendant that went with him on his travels. In the year 1351, King Edward III (1312–1377) paid for hot and cold water for his bathtub at Westminster Palace. Edward had his luxurious bathroom fitted with large bronze taps. The Tudors, especially, were more hygienic than they are given credit for. While they faced the challenges of sewage disposal and bacteria, they did strive to keep themselves, as well as their surroundings, clean. Historians believe that wealthy Tudor women bathed once a day. They were fortunate enough to afford a scented castile soap made from olive oil. Henry VIII was lucky enough to inherit Edward's bathroom at Westminster and made improvements made to several of his other homes. At the Bayne Tower at Hampton Court, Henry had a beautiful bathroom designed with seated windows and a ceiling decorated in gold. The copper bathtubs were supplied with a hot and cold water tap, and a charcoal-fired stove kept the room warm. We aren't sure how often Henry VIII took baths towards the end of his reign due to his increasing size. Still, it has been noted that he was particularly hygienic in his younger days and was repulsed by body odour, especially in women. However, he avoided bathing during outbreaks of sweating sickness or plague. Some thought that washing was quite dangerous and allowed putrid air to enter the body. Although they didn't have the modern-day luxury of the washing machine, Tudors did try to keep their undergarments as clean as possible. It was a sign of respectability. While most nobles tried to change their undergarments once a day, the wealthier may have changed theirs several times a day.

Nobles and monarchs were known for having elaborate dinners and banquets, but this didn't always mean it was healthy. Midday was when dinner was served, which was the biggest meal of the day, consisting of three courses. All three of these courses centred around meat. Boar's head, swan, pheasant, heron, and sturgeon were typical of a first course. Venison, jelly, stuffed pig, peacock, tarts, and fried meat could be enjoyed in the second course. Partridge, quail, pigeon, rabbit, and eggs were served at the final course. While there was undoubtedly a plethora of good food, small samples were usually taken from each session. Spices softened tough meats and preserved them. Spices were seen as representative of a nobles' powers as they were often costly and came from foreign countries.

The lack of refrigeration was probably one of the most significant contributors to foodborne illness, whether you were a noble or not. Fish could usually be caught daily from well-stocked fishponds, and so it wasn't a common problem as long as it was served while still fresh. Meat that had to be stored over winter was dried, smoked, or salted. While

Europe did see some snowy winters, freezing your food was an option but not always. Castles that had cellars could have food packed with ice, but it wasn't terribly common, and there was still the risk that the food wouldn't remain at a safe temperature. Inadequate refrigeration led to listeriosis, which brought about fever, sickness, diarrhoea, and, in rare cases, meningitis. As temperature rises, bacteria grow faster, and this increased the risk of food poisoning.

Contrary to how they are often portrayed, people in the Middle Ages, whether they were from wealthy backgrounds or not, did attempt to eat with clean hands. They usually rinsed their hands in flower water upon rising and before eating. At royal tables, it was not uncommon to share a cup with the person sitting next to you. Because it wasn't easy to get clean drinking water, most meals were served with ale and wine. Of course, sharing a cup with someone was just another way to spread the common cold virus as well as a whole host of infectious diseases.

When we think of the medieval knight, we often picture the iconic soldier in shining armour with his horse, charging into battle with his lance or risking his life to save others. While most of this is true, knights during medieval times didn't have it as luxurious as the storybooks will suggest. Knights served their noble lord, and their lord financed that knight to protect them. They were often granted lands and most probably lived quite comfortably for the times and ate almost as well as their superiors. Knights lived up to a code of chivalry, loyalty, and courage in battle to protect the poor and the weak and be kind to women. Not all knights lived up to this code of honour, but they had been trained to do so. Tales of King Arthur glorified them but being a knight during the Middle Ages was not an easy job.

To become a skilled warrior who could function on horseback while wearing pounds of armour, a boy would start training as a page around seven or eight years of age by learning household chores and good manners. Around the age of fourteen, a page would become an understudy, or squire, of an established medieval knight. He would observe and learn from his master and practice strength training and weapons training. A squire would continue with close combat training, and by the age of twenty-one, he would fulfil his training with an elaborate religious ceremony.

Starting between the year 800 CE and 900 CE, knights were simply warriors on horseback. By the eleventh century, basic armour called chainmail was being used. Chainmail was a type of armour that created a mesh by linking rings of metal together to form a pattern. Eleventh century knights also wore a helmet and carried a sword and lance, which was more like a spear. One problem with wearing chainmail as your only means of defence was that you left yourself open to the enemy's crossbow. The crossbow shot arrows the length of two football fields that could pierce right through chainmail, causing dreadful injury.

Around the 1200s, plate armour was slowly being added to protect the knees and shins of the knight as these were the most vulnerable body parts while on horseback. Over time, a coat was worn over the chainmail with small plates of armour in it. By the 1300s through the 1500s, the plate armour kept piling up until the knight was protected from head to toe. Knights may have been better protected but carrying all that armour around was exhausting. It was estimated that knights wore twenty-five pounds of chainmail and at least fifty pounds of plate armour. If a knight were to be knocked off his horse, it was extremely hard to right himself back up, especially if he were to fall in the water or mud. Such was the case for the French cavalry during the Battle of Agincourt. Once thrown from their horses into the muddy battlefield, most of them were unable to get back up. One of the weapons archers sometimes used in battle was called the longbow, which could shoot between five to twelve arrows in one minute. However, this usually meant that the opposing team also had skilled archers using the same weapon. A direct hit could pierce plate armour and puncture the skin.

Sir William Marshal, Earl of Pembroke (1146–1219), is one of the most renowned knights of the Middle Ages. His proficiency in battle saved the life of Richard I (1157–1199), and he was feared in the jousting tournaments for his skill. William spent his youth training as a squire with the intent of knighthood. He had a reputation as a strong young man with a huge appetite. In 1166, he was knighted and sent almost immediately to action. His early days as a knight showed promise but also the cockiness of an inexperienced warrior. William entered mock cavalry battles and was so impressive that he acquired himself several war horses. He excelled over the next year in tournaments, his wins making himself more profits. During a mock battle where he captured over one hundred knights, his helmet was so severely dented that it got stuck on his head and had to be removed by the local blacksmith.

In 1168, Queen Eleanor (1122–1204), wife of Henry II of England (1154–1189), appointed William to be tutor-in-arms to her fifteen-year-old son. He taught the young prince well, but the Earl of Pembroke was also thought to be sleeping with his wife, Margaret of France (1158–1197). In 1182, William was banished from court. A year later, on the death bed of his former apprentice, they reconciled. He asked William to promise to defend Christendom throughout the kingdom. In 1186, back in battle, William had the future Richard I at his mercy. Richard and his brother John had rebelled against their father, but William chose to spare his life. Such an act was an impressive feat of chivalry. When Richard became king, William was awarded for his kindness. He was betrothed to seventeen-year-old Isabel de Clare (1172–1220), who brought with her a large dowry. William was now a valued member of the court and continued to be so throughout the reign of King John and Henry III (1207–1272). William had honourably served four English Kings and went into battle again in 1217, at the age of seventy, against the future King Louis VIII of France (1187–1226). After a rousing speech to his men, William was victorious in battle once again. William died two years later, and the Archbishop of Canterbury described him as "the greatest knight that ever lived".

The eldest son of Edward III was known as Edward, the Black Prince (1330–1376). While the prince would never sit directly on the throne, he was known as a superb military leader. Edward demonstrated his ability on the battlefield at an early age at the Battle of Crecy in 1346. The prince commanded the right-wing of his father's forces and played a significant role in the English victory at only sixteen years old. Edward III was overcome with emotion after the victory and spoke of the loyalty of his young boy. It was during this battle that Edward obtained the name Black Prince, either because he wore black armour or because his name referred to the cruelty he showed the French during the Hundred Years' War. Edward was appointed his father's lieutenant in 1355, leading another substantial victory against the French, but it was at the Battle of Poitiers in 1356 that Edward won his supreme triumph. He captured Jean II (1319–1364) of France and his youngest son. In 1367, Edward led an expedition into Castile and won a victory in the Battle of Najera. He was significantly awarded by the King of Castile and spend several months in his kingdom. Edward was not a healthy man at times, and it was during the hot summer that he began to exhibit signs of dysentery. A year or so after returning to England on the advice of his physicians, Edward's health declined even further. He spent much time in thoughtful prayer and died peacefully at Westminster in 1376 at the age of forty-five years.

Knights displayed their skills not only on the battlefield but at jousting tournaments. The object of the joust was to capture your opponent, not kill them. But they were using incredibly deadly weapons, including battle axes, maces, and swords made so sharp they could pierce through chainmail. To keep themselves battle-ready, knights had to participate in these tournaments regularly. But this meant continuously putting themselves at risk of horrible wounds, infection, and even death. And on hot days, heatstroke and suffocation were a risk as well. Jousting became most popular throughout the thirteenth century and into the Renaissance. It was a time when nobles and townsmen alike would gather to watch the bravery of knights showing off their battle skills. It was not unheard of for kings to perform in a jousting tournament, although they were putting themselves at risk of death.

One such accident occurred during the reign of Henry VIII in 1536, which is said to have changed his personality significantly. On 24 January at Greenwich Palace, Henry, at forty-four years old, was fully armoured along with his horse, who was also covered in armour. The King was thrown from his horse, and the horse's full weight fell upon him. Unconscious for several hours, his men believed it was a fatal blow for the king. Although he did eventually wake, this was the accident that ended his jousting career and caused an undetected brain injury that profoundly affected his personality. Without the help of modern medicine, it is fascinating to think of what damage the blunt trauma must have done to his brain. It is also amazing to think that he survived without medical intervention.

In June 1559, Henry II of France (1515–1559) was participating in a jousting tournament and was fatally injured. His opponent's lance struck his helmet and pierced through his eye, penetrating his brain. Royal doctors removed the splinter from his eye and his throat, where it had also pierced, but the king continued to bleed profusely and slipped into unconsciousness. The king would succumb to his injuries at just forty years old at the beginning of July.

Knights usually found themselves to be relatively wealthy and lived in more prominent parts of town in townhouses that were often well built, sturdy structures with chimneys and stained-glass windows. Knights also participated in many of the dinners that folks at the top of the feudal ladder did. In doing so, they were lucky enough to partake in the plethora of food available.

If you were the child of a noble or even a knight, you were most likely spared the arduous life of a peasant. At age seven or eight, children of nobles were usually sent away to begin their apprenticeship. Boys could be sent to work as pages in the castle of another lord, where, like knights, they would learn manners and how to dance and play chess. Girls could go to a nunnery if they to were to become a nun. Or they could prepare to marry the man their father selected for them. But either way, children of the upper hierarchy were almost guaranteed a life free from the task of hard labour.

Merchants and craftsmen were considered the middle-class folks of this time, and towns flourished under them. Merchants were almost wholly responsible for the birth and development of the medieval villages and marketplaces. Merchants travelled to lands throughout Europe and Asia to purchase goods and sell them for a much higher price. This travel was often dangerous, harbouring roads that consisted of dirt and mud. They faced treacherous weather, with hardly any inns along the way. They also encountered wild animals and thieves. Merchants needed to learn how to defend themselves, speak other languages, bargain and cheat to survive. Travelling by sea wasn't much different. They were hit with violent storms and pirates who would stop at nothing to steal their goods. The life of a merchant had its risks while travelling, but if you could keep yourself alive, you could make a decent living.

The birth of many towns began when merchants needed a place to store their goods. Wood makers, blacksmiths, bakers, and farmers began heading to town for the opportunity to find work turning these products into valuable assets. Farmers started coming to sell their goods, leeks, beets, carrots, cabbages, apples, eggs, and bread. Butchers brought in live animals, and they were usually slaughtered on the spot for freshness. Over time, these small towns grew into thriving marketplaces with inns and shops. Everything was built by hand, and the jobs of labourers and stonemasons could also be dangerous. While stonemasons made a decent wage, they could easily be crushed by a falling stone. They also made lime mud, which sealed the rocks together. Little did they know, the burning of the lime in their kilns produced carbon monoxide, often causing them to become paralysed. One could easily fall directly into the oven or be overwhelmed by gases. Trade was usually kept in the family and passed down, such as being a weapons maker or a blacksmith.

The primary purpose of the market town was the delivery of goods and services to the locals. In the twelfth century, the number of market towns proliferated. *The Domesday Book*, a manuscript compiled in 1086 by King William I, listed fifty market towns throughout England. The book was a manuscript record of the *Great Survey* of England and parts of Wales. Between 1200 and the year 1349, over 2,000 new towns were constructed across Europe. Market towns were initially close to castles or monasteries because large households would generate the demand for goods. They also offered protection to a market town as a bonus. These towns became the centre of local activity and everyday rural life. English law had established that one marketplace couldn't be within a certain distance of another, usually a day's travel. Over time this created a bit of competition between markets to have the best quality goods. The town strived for a reputation of good produce and foods as well as having the best overnight accommodations for travellers.

Market Harborough is a market town in the district of Leicestershire. A small market had been established in 1204, and it eventually gained the name of Market Harborough. The tradesmen of the marketplace had farms near their property where they were able to produce and store goods. The town steeple was built between 1300 and 1320, and by 1470, much of the town had grown to completion. Blackwell Hall in London became the centre of cloth and wool trade from the Middle Ages through the nineteenth century. It was here at Blackwell that clothing merchants and clothiers would travel to display their material to the public. The market town of Banbury in Oxfordshire was known for its merchants based on the sale and trade of wool.

The majority of market towns in Italy are settled on a hilltop, overlooking a beautiful landscape. *Monte*, meaning *hill* in Italian, is the preface of many of the market towns throughout the country. In the thirteenth century, trade in Italy was on the rise, and the growth of many market towns was at its peak. Montalcino, in Tuscany, was known for its trade in shoes and leather goods. Long periods of prosperity flourished despite many violent episodes in its history. The first walls of the town were built in the early 1300s, and the fortress was erected in 1361. Narrow, short streets branched out from the main gate of the village in beautiful Roman architecture. Montalcino was divided into sections, each with colours to distinguish them. San Gimignano, also in a province of Tuscany, is a small medieval town surrounded by walls. Producers of white wine, San Gimignano families struggled for independence, resulting in over seventy tower houses being built towards the end of the Middle Ages.

France and Germany had their share of impressive market towns as well. Colmar, in France, presents as a picture-perfect medieval village. Beautiful timber houses and weeping willow trees give it a fairy-tale feel. Buildings erected in the fifteenth and sixteenth centuries possess old-world beauty. Colmar was known as a community of wine producers and became known as the region's king of wine. The same old-world feel is prevalent in Nuremberg, Germany. Watchtowers and courtyards stand boastfully in the town. Nuremberg also possesses a dungeon, built in the 1300s, which is an added medieval touch. Rich in the production of bratwurst since the 1300s, the city was also famous for its ale.

No matter which part of Europe you were in, being a craftsman afforded you a higher standard of living above that of a serf or peasant. Homes were respectable and well cared for by the merchant's wife and by a servant or two. But you often found a merchant's house deep within the hustle and bustle of a thriving city or town, and this was not without its problems regarding filth and disease.

Rural peasants and serfs made up the majority of the population during the Middle Ages, and while their day-to-day duties differed very little, there were some differences. Peasants were usually allowed to rent out their lands while serfs lived on the properties of the lords they worked for. Serfs didn't have their freedom, but they weren't precisely slaves. Their lives, like peasants, were built around agriculture. They farmed the lands that the lords provided for them and were able to have their private gardens. The lords offered them protection in return. A peasant, while technically having more rights as a landowner, didn't have the security of a noble lord. Once the decision was made to become a serf, that decision was final. The family was there to stay on the lord's property, while a peasant had the freedom to move about.

The homes of serfs and peasants were much in the same. Called cruck houses, they usually boasted one big room with a bathroom outdoors. They had a wooden frame plastered with a mixture of mud, straw, and manure called wattle and daub. It kept the wind out but offered no protection against intruders. Roofs were built from thatch, consisting of stems, leaves, and grass. Unfortunately, these were also home to bugs and bats. Like the elaborate castles of their lords, the air inside was often thick with smoke from the fireplace. Only they had a fire burning in a much smaller area with much lower ceilings and even less ventilation.

Contrary to modern medicine, there was a belief that smoke was a cure for fever. An added plus was that it covered up body odour. Like the castles, the floors were packed with straw rushes that harboured the same filth and excrement. But rushes also caught the faeces and urine of farm animals, as they were free to wander in and out of homes. At night, animals were brought inside for safety for several reasons. Farm animals were easy prey for the wolves and bears that roamed the forests. The loss of an animal to a peasant would have been disastrous. They also could have been stolen or wandered off, so keeping them inside was the most logical thing to do, but this also had its downfalls. These animals were not house trained, and no doubt added to the unhygienic nature of daily living.

Everyday life was extremely hard for a serf or peasant, as well as for his family. The serf rose at dawn to work the land, every day of the week, except for Sunday. Starting in February, they had to break earth, plough and plant seeds and harvest grain. Usually, boys would help their father in the field as women just weren't strong enough. Women did the cooking and gardening, sewing and caring for the animals and their daughters helped. Everything they ate and more was handmade. It was backbreaking work that was often detrimental to one's health.

Winters were long and cold and proved to be the most challenging time for peasants in the Middle Ages. If there wasn't enough food, one could quickly starve to death, and the risk of contracting pneumonia increased due to the frigid temperatures. Most livestock was eaten over colder months as there wasn't enough to feed them. Homes got incredibly cold, especially at night. Boarded up windows offered little to no sunlight, and people spent much of the winter sleeping as there was little else to do. They slept on wooden pallets, which were narrow, hard mattresses made of straw mixed with scented flowers. Unfortunately, these straw beds attracted bugs, vermin, bed bugs, fleas, and lice. Bed bugs themselves may not have been a transporter of disease, but they inflicted a horrific rash that, when scratched, could undoubtedly lead to a skin infection. And little did people know at the time, but fleas and lice were responsible for the spread of the plague. If they could afford it, they had linen sheets and blankets to provide some warmth against the cold.

Children of serfs and peasants were put to work almost as soon as they could walk. With no promise of an education, there was little choice for them about what lay in their future. By age fourteen, a boy performed all the duties his father did, such as ploughing and harvesting. Girls, by the same age, were doing the same work as their mother. They were expected to cook and weave like their mothers. Life was to work, and all for your lord, if you were a serf. A serf may even be required to fight if his lord went to war, but it would be in situations where they would fight with little or no protection. However, if you worked hard enough, you were usually treated well, with rewards of fish or meat.

Peasant or serf food, although unsavoury, was probably a lot healthier than the diet of nobles and royalty. Breakfast usually consisted of ale and rye bread. Browner bread was more common among peasant folk as white flour was more expensive. If a clean source of drinking water was available, it could be consumed, but it was often hard to come by. The biggest meal came at midday, and because fish was so plentiful, it would usually be salmon along with a sort of pea pottage, as well as bread, beer, and bacon. Supper, being the last meal of the day, was a lighter fare of bread and cheese and ale. And like their noble lords, peasants and serfs did their best to rinse their hands clean before consuming food. But because of their lack of any means of refrigeration, serfs faced an even bigger problem when it came to keeping their food safe for consumption. Veggies that were not kept in appropriate conditions rotted and became infested with vermin. People understood that drying their meats with salt kept them from decaying. But there was still no way around the fact that spoiled food caused great stomach distress. They were under the assumption that parasites originated inside the body and perhaps failed to make the connection between food preparation and illness.

The poor personal hygiene of serfs and peasants was another factor that separated them from those at the top of the feudal system and even from the middle class to some degree. It also significantly contributed to the health of those living in the towns and villages. They simply had no understanding of the connection between hygiene and sickness. Peasants rarely bathed, and some never did at all. With the abundance of waste and no way to deal with it, if they did choose to bath, it was usually in dirty water. Flowers were sometimes used to mask the smell of body odour but most likely did a poor job. There was no running water, of course, this being only for the upper class in extreme cases. Water had to be hauled from rivers, and this required great physical labour. Bathing was done outside, and the water was usually cold. People didn't always use soap but a mixture of lime and salt to clean themselves, which almost certainly caused more inflammation to the skin than anything else. And some just chose not to bother bathing at all, as it was too much effort.

The lack of indoor plumbing throughout homes and towns caused immeasurable filth. Diseases were commonplace, and epidemics decimated towns and villages. About 25% of the population of Europe perished from some sort of disease. Bodily functions were often performed anytime, anywhere, even with public outhouses. In larger cities, the filth and stench were evident almost everywhere. Public baths were standard by the thirteenth century throughout Europe and continued to grow in popularity. Public bathhouses popped up in Paris and along the Thames River in London. Despite their popularity, bathhouses did raise controversy about the fact that men and women saw each other naked. They also became a hotbed for illicit sex and prostitution. The London boroughs of Southwark became famous for its Stews, which were essentially licensed brothels. Not to mention being breeding grounds for disease. The prominence of bathhouses began to decline rapidly into the sixteenth century once people became aware that if you wanted to steer clear of the Black Death and syphilis, it was best to avoid them.

Contrary to popular belief, folks who lived in the Middle Ages were not the toothless and foul breathed people they have been made out to be. Having white teeth and pleasant breath were attributes that many strove for. Sugar wasn't widely available like it is today, and it was also quite costly. It was considered a rare spice and was used primarily for medicinal reasons. Because of the lack of sugar in the early Middle Ages diet, tooth decay wasn't an epidemic like it is now. The production of sugar cane was introduced in the 1500s, and it wasn't until then that it was used in foods. The Tudors had many more problems with tooth decay than those that lived before them. Medieval people did care for their teeth as best they could, even those at the bottom of the feudal ladder. Rough linen or twigs were used to clean the teeth and gums after being dipped in pastes made from salt and sage. Some pastes were mixed with an abrasive and scented herb to freshen breath. Rinses were used as well and made from herbs and spices steeped in wine or vinegar. It was the hard bits of bread and other foods that ground people's teeth down and caused problems. If you did need a tooth pulled, you would usually visit the barber-surgeon, who would happily remove it for you, without anaesthetic, of course.

Because there were no modern bathrooms, you were forced to use the outhouses that were shared with the community. You also had the choice of using a chamber pot, which was then emptied into a cesspit or directly into the river. Cesspits were full of urine, faeces, and garbage, and they contaminated the groundwater and soil to an unimaginable degree.

Serfs usually only owned one set of clothing. Linen was worn next to the skin, and wool was worn over it. Folks in the Middle Ages did understand that washing clothes kept insects away, and they usually washed their clothes once a week in the river with lye soap. The problem was that the river was already polluted with garbage and waste, both human and animal. Fleas and lice were a common problem for most people in the Middle Ages but particularly for people of lower rank. Delousing each other, whether by their fingers or a fine-tooth comb, became an everyday social activity among the town's folks.

As with your role in life, your place on the ladder of society would be indicative of what level of medical care you would expect to receive. Qualified physicians were rare, and many of them had already devoted their efforts to a particular household. Houses of the monarchy or a noble almost always had their own personal doctor. And these doctors usually got paid well, so they made sure they were available when summoned. Often this meant that qualified physicians didn't like to take on extra work as they needed to be available to the highest paying client at all times. The royal household was lucky enough to have a royal surgeon as well as a royal physician, in addition to an apothecary. If you were in a small town or sat at the bottom level of the feudal system, it didn't mean you couldn't get medical care. It just meant that the doctor wasn't likely to be adequately educated. He may not be a doctor at all. He could be the barber-surgeon or simply one who picked up a manual to diagnose patients. Barber-surgeons were aplenty, and usually, folks didn't have too much trouble finding one to carry out some horrific treatment. There was just no promise that you would survive.

I don't believe that people who lived in the Middle Ages were ignorant. I don't feel that you can be ignorant of something that no one truly understood yet. These people had poor knowledge of hygiene and how disease spread. They didn't know about the theory of germs or the way that they multiplied. They also placed so much faith in the divine and believed that God truly was responsible for everything. So perhaps that made it easier for them to be unable to make the connection between their lifestyles and the persistence of disease.

Chapter Four

The Spreading of Disease

In 1796, English physician Edward Jenner (1749–1823) would introduce the vaccine that would help to eradicate smallpox. In the mid to late 1800s, most major European cities rebuilt their sewer systems to modern standards. In 1928, Alexander Fleming (1881–1955) would change the world of medicine with his discovery of antibiotics. But of course, all these brilliant turning points in history were light years away from medieval Europe, where disease ran rampant, and most people lived in absolute squalor.

The bustling cities and towns of the Middle Ages were a far cry from the streets of London or Paris, which today run under strict regulations for cleanliness and order. After the Battle of Hastings and throughout the early fifteenth century, England especially became a place of increasing population. Yet, there was still a lack of knowledge on how to dispose of waste. People had absolutely no idea that they were providing an excellent environment for microscopic killers to thrive.

Roads that led into cities and towns were littered with animal bones and entrails, along with rotted meat thrown about. Human faeces were found next to bushes or, in some cases, right in the road. It was not uncommon to see refuse hauled out by townsmen and tossed into the streams and strewn about the banks. Men would cart barrels of excrement and carelessly throw them into the water. They just didn't understand the horror of what they were doing and saw the rivers and streams as a place to dispose of their waste. All of this garbage came from a place where its people were proud and hardworking, yet also dirty and indulgent. Many of them were utterly filthy, depending on their rank in the feudal society, and reeked of the same stench that came from the sewage rotting alongside the road. If they lived during the reign of a particularly nasty monarch, heads and limbs of executed traitors were on display for all to see, with their rotting eyes having been plucked out by the crows. This unsightly display only added to the filth because it attracted maggots and flies.

Medieval towns were a busy place. Inns and churches, along with merchant's homes and their shops, lined the streets. The marketplace was active, with peasants and local farmers selling their goods. Priests made their way through town, along with workers and their farm animals. Eggs, milk, and cheese were sold to those who desired them. The craftsman's shops were packed tightly together, all offering distinctive goods or trade; blacksmiths, butchers, sculptures, all contributing to the mess and ugliness in the streets. Travellers of all sorts, as well as locals, came in and out of these towns daily to sell and buy goods.

These towns consisted of buildings that varied in shape and size. Some were two or three stories with small alleyways so tiny that they were no more than a few feet across. These houses and buildings were crammed together, sometimes within only four or five feet of each other with little to no sunlight, making the streets dank and overshadowed. Buckets of smelly, rotting food were tossed out of windows to mix in with the churned-up mud and decay laying on the roads. The paths and alleys, boasting no drain systems, became open sewers.

Cities were much the same, just on a larger scale. They were polluted, violent and crowded. There was an overabundance of both people and animals. Vats of water lined the streets in the event of a fire. However, the tubs were usually filled more with decaying rubbish than water. Roads were not paved, and puddles were aplenty. Foul-smelling mud filled the streets, along with animal dung, rotting vegetables, and beast entrails. Rats and dogs were everywhere and just added to the excrement and filth.

Many of these cities, especially London, had an enormous rate of consumption. The suburbs also produced an unrelenting stream of rubbish, animal carcasses, and hides, as most animals were transported alive and slaughtered on sight. Today, descriptions of these places read as if they were the stuff of nightmares or third world countries. But they were really thriving communities built on what were modern conveniences that unfortunately were an open door to death and disease that killed by the thousands.

The rapid development of London began after the Norman invasion in 1066 when William I was crowned king on Christmas Day. Over the next two hundred years, the building of this medieval empire was fast and furious. However, in a place that is now 2000 years old, it was filth that fundamentally shaped the city into what it is today.

William I rebuilt the bridge over the Thames that was initially constructed during the time of the Saxons. The bridge was destroyed by fire in 1091, as this was a constant threat to the city, especially with the construction of wattle and daub buildings. The bridge, rebuilt in 1136, was again consumed by fire. King Henry II created a guild to overlook the rebuilding of the bridge in 1170, and construction was completed in 1209. The bridge was the only way in and out of London over the river, and it swarmed with people, animals, and utter filth. As the population of London began to climb, it became overcrowded with its myriad of high-rise buildings, narrow streets, and merchant's shops that jutted out into the road. Since the Battle of Hastings, the population of the city rose by almost 500%. It is estimated that by the fourteenth century, over 100,000 people were inhabiting the small space between the Thames and the ancient Roman walls of the city. Since 1066, when the grand city was acquired, it had grown considerably. With self-government, London was free. It was a place of escape for serfs and those ruled by the lords of the countryside. It was a place of limitless opportunity. As trade flowed in and out of the Thames, it brought with it the abundance of filth.

Walking through the streets of London meant you had to trudge through sticky, wet mud, along with animal faeces. There were as many people in London as there were animals, and together with the dogs, horses, and pigs, you fought desperately for space. The streets were used as a dumping ground for every kind of refuse one can imagine. Entrails not worthy of eating got tossed into the streets at the hand of the butcher. Chamber pots were dumped out of windows, and people simply walked through the filth. Squalor filled the streets, and because the city government was more concerned with the infrastructure of trade than it was with dealing with sewage, people dealt with it on their own. Wooden shoes called pattens were invented during the Middle Ages and worn over regular footwear. Pattens were held in place by a strap of leather, and they functioned to give you a bit of lift above the muck that filled the streets.

Any accommodations made didn't mean that people weren't getting fed up with the filth that surrounded them on a daily basis. There are records of grievances in the London Metropolitan Archives that state people were starting to file formal complaints. In 1347, there is a case of a townsman who diverted his waste shoot, so it merely emptied into his neighbour's house as a means of avoiding the problem. One woman is also responsible for sending the remnants of her chamber pot right into the rainwater gutters outside her home. The implementation of fines for such things begun in 1309, but it was as if people would rather pay a menial amount of money instead of dealing with their waste. In an attempt to do something about the sewage in the streets, the role of the gong farmer was created towards the end of the fourteenth century. *Gong* was a word used to describe the privy and its contents. While the city had attempted to provide public toilets, the amount available met less than 1% of the population. Cesspits were typically placed under the floor of a home or directly outside the structure. And these cesspits lacked the engineering skills to make them watertight.

Because of this, in addition to the filth in the streets, liquid waste constantly drained from them, leaving more solids to be dealt with, and the gong farmer was brought in to try to contain the growing mess in the city. The amount of waste in the city had grown to over fifty tons a day that had to be disposed of. But digging the debris out of the city streets and cesspits was not only a horrific job, it was downright dangerous. The fumes alone could cause a person to choke to death from asphyxiation. The waste removed was emptied into barrels and loaded onto carts. Because the cesspits of homeowners were typically in their yards, it wasn't uncommon to find things other than food in them. Dead animals and even unwanted infants were sometimes found at the bottom of the pits. Gong farmers would transport the city's waste to the nearby River Thames and dispose of it there. They charged a mighty fee for the job that no one else wanted to do, as much as three times what a regularly paid labourer would cost. Despite the city of London's attempt at controlling the waste problem, it still seemed to be an uphill battle. And uphill was where you wanted to be, because like everything, excretion ran downhill.

As the groundwork for the city continued to be laid, the area grew even more overcrowded. Business may have been booming but at a cost to everyone's health. Excess from city tanners poured into the streets. Being a tanner was a particularly foul job, even to those used to garbage-filled streets. When a tanner acquired the hide of an animal, everything came with it, including manure and blood. Hides were rinsed out directly on the roads, causing more pollution. The animal's hair that was scraped off by the tanner's blade was also dumped into the streets. The hides were washed in chemicals containing urine and lime or fermented rye, causing horrific odours to radiate from them for up to three months. While the job of turning an animal's hide into a material that could be put to good use was admirable, having a tanner working in the streets gave off an awful stink.

Although King Edward II (1284–1327) and his successors may have demanded an abundance of meat in their diets, it didn't change the fact the butchery was also a colossal mess. Pork was popular among royalty, and so the slaughtering of pigs was a common thing. Even while still alive, pigs were a nuisance as they wandered around London. As they were being slaughtered, noxious gasses poured from their bellies into the air. The entrails of the animals were emptied into the streets. If sausage was desired, the stomach linings were at least put to good use. But still, even folks used to the misery of the London streets began to file complaints. In 1343, under the reign of Edward III, butchers were told they needed to dump their waste elsewhere, such as the Fleet River. However, after a time, the river also became overwhelmed with the undesired parts of the animals left after slaughter. Butchers were then directed to the banks of the Thames, but this was a long walk for most. Most became lazy and didn't want to follow the rules as lugging a cart filled with remains through the city took away from their business. But in 1362, the king had had enough and had butchers banned from the city limits, claiming:

> The air of this city is very much corrupted and affected from the putrefied animal blood running down the streets. And the bowels cast into The Thames, whence abominable and most filthy stinks proceed. Sickness and many other evils have become a huge problem in London.

This new law was punishable to those who violated it, and many did. Some butchers were caught selling rotting and putrid meat to the public and suffered the consequences. The offenders were placed in a pillory and forced to inhale the smell of the rotten meat being cooked. The putrid smell was intentionally held underneath their noses for hours at a time.

During the years it took for London to develop, everyone seemed to want to be a part of it in one way or another, and this was the case with other European cities as well. Infrastructure was thriving in Paris, Edinburgh, and Venice, but with the increase in goods and people came a rise in horrific diseases that plagued the Middle Ages throughout its entire existence.

On 10 October 1562, Her Majesty Queen Elizabeth I (1533–1603) fell ill at Hampton Court. She was twenty-nine years old. What was thought to be a bad cold had developed into a violent fever. By 16 October, with her health in severe decline and a rash developing on her hands, the Queen was diagnosed with smallpox. Though it was feared she would die, Queen Elizabeth made a full recovery. But she was left with a plethora of disfiguring scars on her face that she spent the rest of her life trying to cover with lead-based makeup.

Smallpox, caused by the variola virus, was first seen around 10,000 BCE in Africa and found its way to Europe between the fifth and seventh centuries. Doctors discovered that this virus was sudden, as well as contagious, having a fatality rate of around 30%. Smallpox was transmitted through the air and the nasal mucus of those infected. It could also infect another person through bodily fluids or their bedding and clothing. Because of the conditions of the Middle Ages, it is not hard to see how smallpox spread so quickly. The virus first found its way into the mouth and lungs of its victim through inhalation and then to the lymph nodes, where it multiplied and spread to the bloodstream and bone marrow. Those infected would first be struck with a high fever, muscle pain, a general feeling of malaise, headache, nausea, and vomiting. These symptoms would typically last from two to four days. Most physicians were usually able to make a definite diagnosis once the tell-tale rash began to rear its ugly head. Most often starting in the mouth and on the tongue, the smallpox rash would extend over the forehead and face. The extremities became affected, along with the trunk and lower limbs. The spreading of the rash was swift, sometimes taking as little as twenty-four hours.

Smallpox had a few different forms, but because medical literature was not as advanced as it is today, it is believed that the majority of the population affected had ordinary smallpox. In ordinary smallpox, the rash became papules that filled with fluid, called pustules. By the sixth or seventh day, they became raised and embedded into the skin. Fluid slowly leaked from them, and by the second week, they began to dry, forming scabs. After a few weeks, the scabs eventually fell off, usually leaving unsightly scars in their place. In about 5–10% of cases, mostly children, a matter of malignant smallpox would develop. This caused an extremely high fever and severe toxaemia, which was almost always fatal. Haemorrhagic smallpox caused bleeding into the skin, causing it to look charred and black. It was sometimes referred to as the black pox. However, this occurred in less than 2% of adults.

Because medical doctors didn't understand smallpox all that well, the patient was usually provided with supportive care and prayers for recovery. The belief was that smallpox might have been caused by an unhappy deity that was bothered by the colour red. Some of the treatment provided was decorating the room in red. The patient was then wrapped in red sheets as if to draw out the poison caused by the disease. Complications from smallpox, if you survived, could be quite bothersome. Along with pitted scarring, you suffered from respiratory distress. If any of the poxes had been near your eyes, you could suffer from blindness or limited sight.

We know today that it most likely depended on your health whether or not you survived smallpox. It certainly wasn't as disastrous as so many of the other epidemics that tore through Europe in the Middle Ages. Queen Elizabeth had been healthy and was still reasonably young. She had the absolute best medical care one could expect, and so her chances of survival would have been better than anyone else's. Sadly, Elizabeth's friend Lady Mary Sidney, who nursed the queen through her illness, didn't fare as well. Lady Sidney was left horribly disfigured by the disease, so much so that her husband found her almost unrecognizable.

Dysentery, also known as the bloody flux, took the lives of seven monarchs during the Middle Ages. Seven men, who had sat near the top of the feudal system and had all the power of a kingdom at their very fingertips, only to have their lives taken in a most undignified way. In the unsanitary conditions of the Middle Ages, bacteria thrived, and that bacteria known as *shigella* was ruthless. Closely related to E. coli, the effects of shigella have been described in medical text since the time of Hippocrates. Shigella is the bacteria that causes dysentery, very bloody diarrhoea that arose from consuming food and water infected with human faecal matter. Because folks in the Middle Ages didn't understand the importance of proper sewage disposal, it would continuously get mixed in with their drinking water. They certainly understood that drinking water could make you sick; they just failed to know why or how to stop it.

Dysentery caused not only horrific, bloody stools but fever and cramps along with weakness. It also caused dangerous levels of dehydration that were especially fatal to babies under a year old, taking the lives of roughly one third of children before their first birthday. Dysentery preyed on infants and children, and it also tore through armies and cities as well. Bacteria love places where they can multiply, and the filth of a city, as well as the battlefield, would provide ample opportunity for it to do so. But dysentery showed no favourites when it came to social ranking.

King John of England, one of the founders of the Magna Carta, is remembered for his ill-temper and distasteful ways with women. John was the third king in the House of Plantagenet and the youngest of four sons of King Henry II of England. He had become his father's favourite after his brothers revolted against the king. John gained the crown after the death of his brother Richard in 1199. King John was cocky, dangerous, and war hungry. Pope Innocent III (1161–1216) also excommunicated him in 1209. He quickly gained a reputation as a cruel ruler who overlooked the rules of the Kingdom. He alienated his country by raising taxes and treated his nobles heartlessly, being known as a sexual predator with their wives and daughters. King John also starved people to death, even children. In September 1216, while England was deep in civil war, he contracted dysentery in the town of King's Lynn. He moved west but continued to weaken. The king had been on the move and was under a great deal of strain. Battlefield living conditions were most likely filthy and primitive. And for a person who was both physically and emotionally exhausted, he was a target for the misery of dysentery. By the time he reached Newark Castle, he was too sick to go any further. He fell victim to dysentery on 18 or 19 October, either sitting directly on the toilet trying to have a bowel movement or very close to it.

King John was just one of several monarchs to succumb to dysentery. His brother, Henry the Young King (1155–1183), was the titular King of England and son of Henry II. Although he held no real power and wasn't terribly interested in government, he still held great importance due to his bloodline. At age 28, while pillaging local monasteries, he contracted dysentery and died on 11 June. Louis IX of France (1214–1270), who was the only King of France to be granted sainthood, also lost his life to dysentery. Louis IX played an active part in the seventh and eighth Crusades, and when the bacteria tore through his army in August 1270, he was not spared. Edward I of England (1239–1307) was known as a temperamental, intimidating monarch who spent much of his reign in turmoil with Scotland's Robert the Bruce (1274–1329). During retaliation against the Scottish king, Edward I developed dysentery just south of Scotland's border. On 6 July 1307, he fell directly into the arms of one of his servants and died. Philip V of France (1293–1322), who played an essential role in the crusade movement as well as being involved in the politics of the Leper Scare of 1321, died of dysentery at Longchamp Abbey in Paris. Henry V of England (1386–1422) was also known for his outstanding military success during the Hundred Year War. He is remembered for his valour during the Battle of Agincourt. It is believed that he, too, succumbed to dysentery on 31 August 1422 and died quite suddenly.

It's ironic to think that something unseen by the naked eye could so weaken so many men of such military greatness and strength. Imagine knights in plated armour, charging into battle one minute, only to be left holding their bellies over the privy the next.

Cholera was yet another bacterial infection of the intestine that brought with it severe, profuse, watery diarrhoea and vomiting. The bacteria *Vibrio Cholerae* was responsible for the illness that also caused rapid heart rate and dry mouth, and restlessness in children. Like dysentery, cholera was found in the faeces of an infected person. The disease quickly spread through the areas of inadequate sewage and drinking water and became an epidemic throughout the Middle Ages. People were contagious as soon as six hours to as long as seven to fourteen days from being exposed.

Reports of cholera-like illnesses have been found in India as early as 1000 AD and are thought to have affected humans for centuries. Like many of the epidemics that ravaged cities and towns, medieval doctors were convinced that cholera was caused by a miasma or an atmosphere polluted by air or decaying bodies. The severe dehydration caused by cholera often led to renal failure and electrolyte imbalance, coma, shock, and death in as few as eighteen hours. The mortality rate was as high as 50–60% because doctors just didn't understand that rehydration would have made a world of difference in their patient's chance of survival.

By the Tudor period, the Stews had infamously become a place of ill repute and vile behaviour. They became brothels and a perfect place to share the gift of syphilis.

The primary thought process behind the rise of syphilis was that it was carried to Europe from the Americas as a product of the Columbian Exchange. It was well recorded in 1495 among the French troops of King Charles VIII (1470–1498) and believed to have been transmitted to them through Spanish mercenaries. But there is also evidence that suggests that syphilis may have existed in Europe as early as the 1300s. Skeletal remains found at the Augustinian Friary in Hull in the United Kingdom show signs of syphilis such as pockmarks and destructive lesions in the bone. Both are classic cases of syphilis.

While today it is still debatable how exactly syphilis reached Europe, there was no question at the time that this bacterium was a significant killer during the Renaissance and was sexually transmitted. The people understood that intercourse caused syphilis and that prostitution bore the brunt of it. And the stews of Southwark were ripe with prostitutes. People realised that once a prostitute was infected, they then passed it onto a new client, who gave it to another woman, maybe even his wife, and it became a deadly circle. Syphilis also became incredibly stigmatised due to its nature of being a sexually transmitted disease. The bacteria *Treponema Pallidum,* known as syphilis, that would wreak absolute havoc over Europe, came in three stages.

In the first stage of the disease, one would find themselves with weeping, although painless, genital sores called chancres. The second stage of syphilis would begin about three to six months after infection, and the patient would present with a genital rash, which would eventually spread over the body. Flu-like symptoms would arise, and the victim would notice warts in their mouth as well as their genitals. This stage of the disease was the most contagious and could last a few weeks to a year. It was the third stage of syphilis that caused considerable damage. Elevations on the skin continued, followed by infections in the skin, swelling, and paralysis. Nerve pain was often accompanied by heart attacks. A feeling of going insane and a great feeling of shame engulfed the individual. The final stage of syphilis also caused ulcerations on the face, and people looked as if their flesh was eaten off the bone, often with their nose caving in. Tumours would grow all over the body and creep into the nervous system, causing seizures and dementia.

Doctors and clergy alike believed that syphilis was the wrath of God, an apparent punishment for the immoral acts of sinners. And the people of every country that syphilis affected blamed its spread on the foreigners of another country. The word syphilis derives from a poem written by Italian physician and mathematician Girolamo Fracastoro (1478–1553) entitled *Sive Morbus Gallicus*. Syphilis means the "French Disease".

German physician Joseph Grunpeck (1473–1532), whose writing has been well documented, called syphilis, the French Evil. He writes:

> Above all these punishments, there has arisen a previously unheard of, unseen, unknown to all mortals, a dreadful, stinking, pimply, and disgusting sickness with which people are being severely stricken, the like of which has never before appeared on earth.

When Grunpeck himself became infected, he described the disease as "so cruel, so distressing, so appalling that until now nothing more terrible or disgusting has ever been known on this earth". He went on to explain, "the wound on my priapic gland became so swollen, that both hands could scarcely encircle it".

Whether they picked it up from Spanish mercenaries or if it was in Europe long before, it was clear that when Charles VIII of France (1470–1498) led his troops into Northern Italy in August 1494, they brought more than an army of men with them. After seizing Naples, the French soldiers had an extended celebration in a city that was already rich with brothels and disease. Upon returning to their homeland at the end of 1495, syphilis would spread through France, Switzerland, and Germany. It would reach England and Scotland in 1497. The Holy Roman Emperor Maximillian I of Austria (1459–1519) proclaimed that nothing like this disease had ever been seen before and that it was a punishment from God.

People who encountered syphilis were terrified of it and even more so than the plague. They had heard the tales of the plague and how it had wiped out almost half of Europe. But the Black Death had done so quickly. Syphilis stuck with you for years and slowly drove one insane. Syphilis earned the name *The Great Pox*, and the impact it had on Europe was devastating. As infected populations grew, popular targets of strict laws were often the beggars and sex workers. Paris ordered all the beggars to leave the city so they could starve to death in the country. Sex workers that went near anyone in the army would have their noses and ears slit. Foreigners thought to have syphilis were asked to leave whatever country they were visiting. Like most epidemics of the Middle Ages, syphilis didn't choose its victims. Even the wealthy were affected. If the wealthy were infected, they were confined to their homes and asked not to leave. The poor were sent to hospitals and usually publicly whipped to shame them. Anyone disobeying these rules could be executed depending on the country's laws. In Paris, if you didn't leave the city when asked, you risked being drowned in the Seine River. Once it reached Scotland in 1497, Edinburgh began to close its brothels. At the beginning of the 1520s, Henry VIII of England grew extremely concerned about prostitution and began to close the stews and bathhouses as he ordered regulations put in place.

The sweating sickness has always been a disease that has especially interested me. Perhaps it is because of the velocity at which it took its victims, or maybe it is because it was considered a disease of the Tudors. Whatever the reason, I feel that the sweating sickness doesn't get the recognition it deserves and is often overshadowed by its more well-known counterparts. But if you lived in the fifteenth century, with its mortality rate between 30–50%, the sweating sickness was terrifying.

Known as The Sweat or English Sweat because it was recorded to only claim victims of English descent, its first outbreak was in 1485 during the War of the Roses. Some believe that the sweating sickness may have come from French mercenaries that were part of Henry Tudor's army at the Battle of Bosworth. After claiming his throne, Henry arrived in London on 19 September 1485, and by October, the English sweat had killed almost 15,000 people. French physician, Thomas Forrestier, who was living in London, noted on 19 September 1485:

> We saw two priests standing together and speaking together and saw both of them die suddenly. Also, in proximity, we see the wife of a tailor and suddenly died. Another young man walking by the street fell down suddenly. Also, another gentleman riding out of the city died. Also, many others the which to rehearse we have known that have died suddenly.

Doctors weren't sure exactly what caused sweating sickness, but they knew it was highly contagious. Possibly it was again from poor sanitation and contaminated water. Experts today believe that the sweating sickness was probably a form of hantavirus, a pulmonary syndrome mainly found in Europe and Asia. What's interesting is that while so many other epidemics of the Middle Ages seemed to affect the lower classes, the sweating sickness seemed to claim England's upper class as its victims.

The sweat started quite suddenly with a feeling of anxiety, followed by shivers and an intense headache. Pains in the neck and the legs took over the patient, along with utter exhaustion. This was referred to as the cold stage and lasted anywhere from half an hour to three hours. The hot stage followed, which was an overwhelming feeling of heat and sweating that overtook the body. The person broke out in a sweat for no reason, almost in a heat delirium with an increased pulse and an insane thirst. The final stage of the disease, if you survived, was sheer exhaustion.

The quickness that the sweating sickness struck with was terrifying. It seemed to strike at night or early morning and would leave doctors scrambling for optimal treatment. Often methods to save patients contributed to their mortality. It appears as if the acuteness of the sweat lasted roughly twenty-four hours, and you either survived or you didn't. In some cases, people died in only a few short hours. In 1517, Chronicler Edward Hall wrote, "this malady was so cruel that it killed some within three hours, some within two hours, some merry at dinner and dead at supper".

The sweating sickness hit England again in 1507, killing 91 people in three days. It is also believed that Prince Arthur Tudor (1486–1502), son of Henry VIII, may have lost his life to sweating sickness in April of 1502. In 1517, Thomas Cromwell (1485–1540), a lawyer and member of parliament who had lost his wife and daughter to sweating sickness, expressed concern that it was killing members of the royal household. Cardinal Thomas Wolsey, a prominent figure of Henry VIII's Privy Council, is said to have contracted the disease more than once and survived. However, he lost fifteen members of his household in 1517. The illness returned again in 1528, where it grabbed hold of the English court and affected over 40,000 people in London. It started in the capital city in May of that year and quickly spread throughout England with an extremely high mortality rate. King Henry VIII, who already had an unhealthy paranoia of illness, broke up his court and left London, frequently changing his residence. In June, the king's mistress Anne Boleyn came down with the sweating sickness and almost died. Many other nobles got sick, and several died. And in 1551, it returned yet again, killing nearly 1,000 in London by July alone. Henry Machyn, a tailor who provided clothing and other articles for funerals in the city, cited in his diary, "On the 7th of July began a new sweat in London".

In 1552, after the epidemic of the sweat seemed to have left, English physician John Caius (1510–1573) published a source of clinical information called *Sweate*. His description is as follows:

> This disease is not a Sweat only (as it is thought and called), but a fever, as I said, in the spirits by putrefaction venomous ... First, by the pain in the back or shoulder, pain in the extreme parts, as arm, or leg, with a flushing, or wind, as it seems too certain of the patients, feeling in the same ... Secondly by the grief in the liver and the nigh stomach. Thirdly, by the pain in the head, & madness of the same ... Fourthly by the passion of the hart ... Whereupon also follows a marvellous heaviness, (the fifth token of this disease), and a desire to sleep, never contented, the senses in all parts being as they were bound or closed up, the parts, therefore, left heavy, vanished, and dull ... Last follow the short abiding, a certain Token of the disease.

Even today, the English sweat remains an epidemiological mystery. It seems to have disappeared almost entirely by late Elizabethan times. While most have agreed that it was a form of *hantavirus*, medical experts speculate that the virus may have mutated to a less infectious strain or that it became much more fatal to its rodent hosts. Another thought is that it may have changed along with the climate. Europe was becoming increasingly colder, especially towards the end of the Tudor era. The change in weather may have made it harder for the disease to survive and spread.

Named after the monks of the order of St. Anthony, St. Anthony's Fire is one of the lesser-known outbreaks of the Middle Ages, but one I feel deserves mention because of its peculiarities. St. Anthony's Fire was the name given to a madness that was caused by a fungus called ergot, which grows on ryegrass. The fungus contaminated the rye flour used in baking. Ergot caused vivid hallucinations in people causing them to writhe in agony or run in the streets. People were said to vomit and feel like they were being burned at the stake. Ergot contains ergotamine, which in small doses is used today to treat haemorrhaging patients or to promote contractions in birthing mothers. But in large doses, it can be disastrous. Ergot paralyzes the nerve endings, causing pain and gangrene of the hands and feet as the blood supply is restricted.

King Magnus II of Norway (1048–1069) died from St. Anthony's Fire shortly after the Battle of Hastings in 1066. Having ruled for only three years, King Magnus was thought to have died from ringworm. Modern historians, however, have proposed that it was ergotism. It's hard not to have sympathy for King Magnus when the phases of death from ergotism sound atrocious. Especially because he was remembered as "an amiable king and bewailed by the people". Judging from detailed writings of death by ergotism, King Magnus likely suffered from painful convulsions. Excruciating spasms, together with diarrhoea, headaches, nausea, and vomiting, were also said to include mania and psychosis. The stages of gangrene that followed were probably a result of the narrowing blood vessels caused by the alkaloids in the ergot fungus. Toes and fingers were most often affected, along with the loss of sensation and eventually the dying off of tissue.

There isn't too much more mention of St. Anthony's Fire in history other than what is known as the Dancing Plague of 1518. In Strasbourg, Alsace, which is today modern France, there was an epidemic in 1518, known as a dancing mania. Almost 400 people, primarily women, danced themselves into a frenzy, some to the point of death. It started with one woman in July and quickly escalated to around 400. Physicians didn't understand why but many of these women danced themselves to death. Some had heart attacks or strokes; some collapsed and died from sheer exhaustion. Physicians at the time ruled out any astrological or supernatural causes. They decided that it was a congenital disease that was caused by *hot blood*. Modern theory today suggests that it was caused by food poisoning. The chemical responsible being the products found in ergot fungi, which is closely related to lysergic acid diethylamide or LSD. It certainly makes sense if you think about how these women danced themselves into absolute madness, as modern descriptions of LSD usage are similar.

Few diseases during the Middle Ages have evoked the kind of social response that leprosy has. Leprosy was both misunderstood and feared. It was seen as a curse from God, and lepers were often stigmatised and shunned. The many misconceptions about this disease were again due to the simple lack of education that medical doctors had.

Leprosy is an infectious disease, a bacterium called *mycobacterium leprae*. But contrary to the beliefs of medieval doctors, it wasn't contracted that easily. It became known as Hansen's Disease after the bacteria was discovered by Norwegian doctor Armauer Hansen (1841–1912) in 1873. Historians believe that leprosy was around during the time of the ancient Greeks, as Hippocrates does talk about it in 460 BCE. Alexander the Great's (356 BCE–323 BCE) soldiers are believed to have contracted leprosy during their campaign in India, where it was eventually brought to the Mediterranean and spread slowly to Europe. It is recorded to have reached epidemic proportions in the fourth century and then again in the Middle Ages, beginning around 1100. It was around this time, after the Norman Conquest, that leper hospitals began to pop up around London.

Although it wasn't as contagious as other bacteria, experts believe that leprosy was caused by poor living conditions, poor diet, and close contact. It was spread through mucus droplets from the nose and mouth but usually took three to twenty years to show the first signs that you were infected. The early symptoms of leprosy started with skin lesions and decreased sensation. Muscle weakness and numbness of the hands and feet would follow. People often complained of problems with their eyesight along with nose bleeds. Their fingers would begin to curl, which was caused by paralysis of the hands. Ulcers would start to appear on their feet. Because of the lack of feeling, the patient was more prone to injuries and breaks. A patient could repeatedly damage appendages and lose them due to decreased blood flow. Wounds became infected because of a weakened immune system, and tissue began to break away. The mucus membranes began to deteriorate, and one's nose could easily collapse. The nerves responsible for blinking would become destroyed over time, and a person would be left unable to blink, leading to eye infection and blindness. Leprosy permanently damaged the skin, causing a person to become deformed for the rest of their lives.

Physicians had to take great care in making an accurate diagnosis of leprosy because a definite diagnosis was life-altering. Once it had been decided that you were to be admitted into a leper hospital, arrangements were then made to get all of your personal affairs in order. One could expect that life would never be the same after a diagnosis was made. Leprosy was a significant health concern, and some communities went to great lengths to protect themselves. While some did treat lepers with compassion, most were socially isolated. People were indeed weary of lepers, but they weren't wholly looked at as people who should be alienated from society. There is a large misconception that has been drawn by physicians well past the Middle Ages that lepers were utterly ostracised. However, these misconceptions are generally unfounded. Only about 10% of leprosy victims reached the point where their body parts would fall off or lead to disfigurement. While it may have been distressing to townspeople to witness the disease, most did not resort to shunning them. As I will explain in a later chapter, it was primarily nineteenth century art that gives us the idea that society wanted nothing to do with lepers. In extreme cases, their voices became hoarse, and they would stagger about like corpses. This behaviour probably instilled fear into the town's people.

Leprosy affects the larynx, damaging mucus and sensory nerves that often resulted in aspiration. Oedema eventually evolves, and nodules develop on the larynx. This is typically manifested through the loss of one's voice, causing lepers sometimes to carry a bell to warn others of their presence in the event they could not speak. But again, it was a lack of understanding into the later 1800s regarding the disease that sparked unnecessary outcry. It was in the 1200s that the law *Ludicium Leprosorum*, which was a judgment of the lepers, gave the condition more of a medical recognition. Doctors were paid by the state to inspect the bodies of folks suspected of being lepers so the court could decide whether or not they should be sent to a leper hospital. This procedure of judgment took place in many different parts of Western Europe from the early thirteenth century.

Along with medical practitioners, parish priests, civil officials, and administrators from leper hospitals could all be present for the event. It was a collaborative diagnosis, but the various parties may have differed in their findings. It was often the case between doctors and lawyers and the layman of the community.

Lepers were at risk of being some of the most abused people during the Middle Ages. Because it was believed that their disease was contagious, they were almost constantly denied entry into settlements. In 1321, an alleged conspiracy of fed-up French lepers that intentionally poisoned water supplies and wells with powders and poisons became known as *The 1321 Leper's Scare*. The plot flourished after the Shepherds Crusade of 1320, an attack on Jews in France. In retaliation, powders made with contaminated bread were used to pollute the water. Bernardo Gui, (1261–1331) papal inquisitor, writes:

58   Medicine in the Middle Ages

In 1321, there was detected and prevented an evil plan of the lepers against the healthy persons in the kingdom of France. Indeed, plotting against the safety of the people, these persons, unhealthy in body and insane in mind, had arranged to infect the waters of the rivers and fountains and wells everywhere, by placing a poison and infected matter in them and by mixing (into water) prepared powders, so that healthy men drinking from them or using the water thus infected, would become lepers, or die, or almost die, and thus the number of the lepers would be increased and the healthy decreased. And what seems incredible to say, they aspired to the lordship of towns and castles, and had already divided among themselves the lordship of places, and given themselves the name of potentate, count, or baron in various lands, if what they planned should come about.

As mentioned before, the iconic picture of the leper being shunned from society wasn't entirely accurate. Lepers were also looked at in Christendom as someone whose trials brought them closer to earning the salvation of Jesus Christ. They were the ultimate symbol of the poverty of Christ. A pivotal moment in the life of St. Francis of Assisi (1181–1226) is when he embraced his fear of the leper and found himself living among them and caring for them. St. Francis was born in 1182 and was known as a carefree young man with dreams of becoming a knight. Like many in his social circle at the time, Francis avoided lepers as he felt disgusted by them. He credited God himself for changing his mind on the day he caught sight of a leper on the road. Although his instincts were to turn away in revolt, Francis instead embraced the man. The leper's hands had begun to rot away from an extreme case of the disease, but Francis felt no fear as he held the man's hands in his own. Francis saw this man as a representative of Jesus Christ. In his testament of the event, he wrote:

> When I was in sin, the sight of lepers nauseated me beyond measure, but then God himself led me into their company, and I had pity on them. When I had once became acquainted with them, what had previously nauseated me became a source of physical consolation for me. After that, I did not wait long before leaving the world.

Francis soon dedicated his life to caring for the lepers as Christ would have. He understood that his mission in life was to serve the most unfortunate of humankind. His acts of compassion are believed to have shown people throughout time that caring for the poor was the path to salvation.

In the course of human history, the Black Death, or the Black Plague, remains one of the most devastating pandemics of all time. It caused complete religious, social, and economic upheaval and forever changed Europe. Also known as the Pestilence, the Black Death was responsible for an estimated 40 to 50 million deaths throughout Europe and Asia between the years 1347 and 1351.

During the beginning of 1348, people in Europe felt secure under the feudal system. They knew where they stood, and cities were flourishing under what was a kind and merciful God. However, at the beginning of that same year, rumours were starting to swirl about a growing catastrophe in the eastern part of the world. Merchants who travelled to Asia came back to Europe with stories of what sounded like a time of absolute doom; fire breathing dragons and serpents were falling from the sky and tearing into the flesh of the innocent.

It's not possible to pinpoint the exact area that the Black Death arose from, but some theories give us a general idea. It made its initial appearance in the Crimean Peninsula in 1347, but its origins go back even further. The city of Caffa, a trading post near the Black Sea, was operated by merchants from the Italian city of Genoa. Caffa dominated trade and had become a major seaport and home to one of Europe's largest slave markets. But the city was also under a military blockade under the Mongolian Army. The Italian merchants soon learned that the army surrounding their city had come down with a strange and deadly illness. The leader of the Mongols, Jani Beg, needed a way to get rid of the bodies of his army that were piling up. He also realised he had a way to spread the devastating disease to the people of Caffa. While the Mongols were practising Muslims, the Genoese merchants were Christian. The religious differences between the two resulted in previous disputes that continued to grow into hatred. Historians agree that the Black Death had been ravaging Central Asia since 1331. It was carried by fleas that travelled on the bodies of rats. The rodents had migrated from Asia's famine-stricken land to the Crimean Peninsula. By the time the Mongols had begun their siege on the city of Caffa, they were struck down by fever, with lumps arising on their bodies and dead skin on their faces. As army commanders watched the plague tear through their men, they saw it as a way to give Caffa a taste of the deadly and mysterious disease. The bodies of the dead were set on catapults and flung over the intimidating walls of Caffa. The townspeople of Caffa watched in horror as rotting corpses fell from above, spreading their infection throughout the city. The people tried in desperation to move the bodies into the sea, but they were too late, for the Black Death had already taken hold. Italian merchants who survived the bizarre sickness fled west to Italy.

In January 1348, as boats from Caffa began to dock in Genoa, other ships had already reached the shores of Sicily in October 1347. People were starting to get very sick as the plague spread like wildfire. This was the start of a disease that would utterly ravish humanity. It soon reached the shores of Venice and Pisa in only a few weeks before it began to sweep across Europe.

In autumn 1347, the ports of northern Italy were bustling with trade. What the people didn't see coming was the utter devastation that was lurking on the ships coming into port, with sailors returning from Caffa and the Black Sea in the east. These sailors were already sick with the plague. Gabriel de Mussis (1280–1356), an Italian notary, who recorded some of the most detailed writings of the epidemic in Italy, described it as such:

> When the sailors reached these places and mixed with the people there, it was as if they had brought evil spirits with them: every city, every settlement, every place was poisoned by the contagious pestilence, and their inhabitants, both men, and women, died suddenly. And when one person had contracted the illness, he poisoned his whole family even as he fell and died, so that those preparing to bury his body were seized by death in the same way. Thus, death entered through the windows, and as cities and towns were depopulated, their inhabitants mourned their dead neighbours.

Italian cities would soon be on the brink of destruction in what was the most remarkable human catastrophe of mankind.

The plague appeared to come in two separate components. The pneumonic form began with a fever and vomiting and a general flu-like feeling, and possible spitting of blood. In the bubonic phase, a swelling would start in the neck, groin, or armpits, eventually forming a bubo.

The bubo was the tell-tale sign of the plague. These swollen lymph nodes could develop from the size of an egg to a small apple. Internal haemorrhaging under the skin would produce black blotches signifying that death was usually soon to follow. Within a week, the victim would die from flooding of the lungs. The Black Death had been given its name due to the necrosis of skin cells on the body. The skin turned black even while the victim was still alive, and it was almost inevitable that one had to witness their own decomposition while still alive. Folks saw the burned appearance of themselves and their loved ones as a sign of the end of life as they knew it.

Italian writer Giovanni Boccaccio (1313–1375), who lived through the plague, had written detailed accounts of the disease in his book, *The Decameron*. He gave a graphic description of what he saw in Italy:

> The symptoms were not the same as in the East, where a gush of blood from the nose was the plain sign of inevitable death; but it began both in men and women with certain swellings in the groin or under the armpit. They grew to the size of a small apple or an egg, more or less, and were vulgarly called tumours. In a short space of time, these tumours spread from the two parts named all over the body. Soon after this, the symptoms changed, and black or purple spots appeared on the arms or thighs or any other part of the body sometimes a few large ones, sometimes many little ones. These spots were a certain sign of death, just as the original tumour had been and still remained.

Within two to three months, 20% of the population of northern Italy was dead, and doctors had absolutely no idea how to stop it from continuing. Gentile da Foligno (1280–1348), the chief physician at the University of Perugia, said it was worse than anything he had ever seen. Fear had gripped the country as people watched the plague take down people of every rank and creed.

Caused by the bacteria *yersinia pestis*, the Black Death, like many other conditions of the time, was believed to come from bad air. This belief, the Miasma Theory, was an archaic medical theory that suggested diseases like the Black Death or cholera were literally caused by pollution or something terrible in the air.

As the plague tore through the seaside towns and moved inland, it wreaked absolute havoc on the country. Highly contagious, the disease killed in as little as two to three days. The sick would spread it to anyone who came near them. Even to touch the clothes of the sick or anything else they came in contact with would almost guarantee you would become unwell. The medical profession felt they were helpless and offered little relief for the symptoms. They couldn't be sure if one became infected by the air, food, touch, or all of the above. As the disease progressed, everything the body excreted came with an overpowering smell. Whether it was sweat, or faeces, or even a person's breath, everything smelled of rot. Bodies, some not even dead yet, would be carried away by coffin bearers. Coffin bearers were usually folks at the very bottom of society, sometimes even criminals, who looked for bribery to carry off corpses. Bodies were sometimes left in the streets if the family was too poor to afford a funeral. The dead would then be thrown in a communal pit. Bodies were also brought to churches by the hour for burial. Because there was just not enough land, they were buried in trenches by the thousands. People saw this devastation as the wrath of God and believed they were being punished for their sins

The efforts to provide relief by da Foligno, such as applying a paste made from dried excrement and white lily to the buboes, proved fruitless. The act of rubbing a hot onion on the buboes probably didn't harm the patient any further, but it surely didn't provide a cure. Doctors were desperate to try anything. Patients had put their faith in God and in their doctors, who sometimes refused to visit. And although da Foligno stood out as going to great lengths to help his patients, he too fell victim to the plague on 18 June 1348.

By this time, death in Italian cities had skyrocketed. Venice had lost over 90,000, and Florence, over half its population. In Sienna, victims were tossed over the city walls into pits, left to pile on top of each other. Houses were ordered to be locked in Milan, and infected people were left to die.

According to a fourteenth century chronicle written by the Grey Friars at Lynn, the plague arrived in Dorset, England, in early May 1348. The first major city to be struck was Bristol, and by late September, it had reached London. The filth of the Southwark brothels made it an open invitation for the disease. The devastation throughout the city was horrific. The transmission of the plague thrived on busy, dirty streets with overcrowded and unsanitary conditions. Authorities struggled to keep up disposal of the corpses but found that the street cleaners were quickly dissipating faster than they could be employed. The burial grounds of London were overflowing, and new ones were carelessly dug. In Southwark alone, an estimated 200 bodies were disposed of daily. Bodies were thoughtlessly piled on top of one another in an attempt to save space. Or worse, older bodies were dug up and moved to make room for the newly deceased. With such immense pressure put on graveyard workers, speed was the only factor. There was hardly time for prayer or the blessings of a priest.

By March 1349, the plague began its descent onto southern England, spreading into rural villages by spring. Entire families were wiped out, and death was imminent. The epidemic ripped through communities, killing over 700 people in only a few months. Many villages lost almost 80% of their population, paralyzing their way of life. In Paris, the disease took nearly 800 people a day. All over Europe, the plague caused a complete breakdown of society. Boccaccio wrote:

> One citizen avoided another; hardly any neighbour troubled about others, relatives never or hardly ever visited each other. Moreover, such terror was struck into the hearts of men and women by this calamity, that brother abandoned brother, and the uncle his nephew, and the sister her brother, and often the wife her husband. What is even worse and nearly incredible is that fathers and mothers refused to see and tend their children, as if they had not been theirs.

The enforcement of laws began to dissipate because its enforcers were either dead or had shut themselves up in their homes in fear of catching the plague. People looked for any way to fight the disease. Citizens of London began to wall themselves in the city in the hopes of keeping the epidemic at bay. But this only caused it to spread more, for it thrived on an atmosphere of close contact and filth. Venice had issued a quarantine for all ships arriving into its ports, but it was already too late for them as well. Milan had just about shut everyone out of the city entirely. To find a way to cover up the stench of rotting corpses, people doused themselves in heavy perfume. They believed that if the cause were bad air, they would be able to keep from getting sick if they didn't breathe in the stench. People kept their windows shut and changed their diets, anything they thought worthy of helping to protect them. And unlike the lepers from earlier in the century, plague victims were generally looked at with absolute horror. Those that were wealthy enough would flee Europe's capital cities, but the poor stayed in the cities and brothels. The attitude soon became that if you were going to die, why not do it with a smile on your face. Folks unashamedly abandoned their morals. Cities became full of drunkenness and illicit sex. Homes were pillaged and goods taken without asking. The Black Death had torn through the bonds of faith and trust between people and their communities.

Priests, too, grew scared to visit the sick and with good reason. In Piacenza, the plague devastated a religious order where over fifty priests died. It was estimated that the mortality rate for priests during the Black Death was over 40%. As the plague scourged across Europe and reached southern France, it spread to the papal seat of Avignon. Pope Clement VI (1342–1352), who was considered to be God's voice on earth, sat on the papal throne. The Church believed that it was a wind deity that brought the pestilence to the people because of their moral decent. It was God's way of punishing people. The Pope affirmed that it was prayer that would lead people to salvation. He was wrong. The Avignon Papacy lost one third of its cardinals and half of its population. Many felt, in a time of great peril, that the Catholic Church was failing them.

Some answers as to why the plague had come were found in the stars. Astrologers believed that God had caused the planets to line up in a way that brought about the disease. Others thought that he had caused great earthquakes that released deadly gases that rose from the ground to punish his people. Folks turned their prayers to the saints. Saint Sebastian (256–288) was looked at as a saint who could intervene on people's behalf and protect them from the plague. The devotion to him increased dramatically but to no avail.

In response to the disgruntlement with the Church, a group of religious zealots began to make an appearance. This religious sect called themselves the Flagellants and stepped up to challenge the authority of the pope. They believed they would receive atonement for their sins by vigorously whipping themselves in public. They journeyed through Europe thirty-three days at a time, one day for each year that Christ walked the earth. Processions through the streets of major cities were led by both men and women, barefoot and covered in ashes. They chanted and performed bizarre rituals. Wearing hoods with red crosses, they repeated litany as they beat themselves with whips, marching from town to town. They saw themselves as representatives of Jesus suffering on the cross and drew in large crowds of people. The opposition infuriated the Church as it was done without their authority. They believed the flagellants to be fanatics who did nothing but spread the plague to even more people with their filth and spattered blood. And the flagellants also spread hate and bigotry as they blamed the Jews for the horror of the plague. Entire villages of Jews were burnt down, especially in parts of Germany. Panic over the Black Death turned to acts of savagery, as the imaginations of the Germans told them that the Jews were to blame. Rumours began to spread that the Jews had poisoned the wells of their neighbours in an attempt to infect others. While this wasn't the case, enough Jews confessed under torture. And once these "confessions" reached the cities of Germany, chaos began. In cities such as Munich and Stuttgart, in November 1348, Jewish cities were burned beyond recognition.

When the plague began to ravage the city of Avignon, physicians began to flee the city, but Guy de Chauliac (1300–1368), a papal surgeon, stayed to document symptoms of the disease in meticulous detail. While treating others, he contracted the disease himself and miraculously survived. It is considered that he excised the buboes from his body himself. After he recovered, he worked tirelessly to help others. His accounts gave fascinating details of the horror of the plague. He reported to the papal court:

> The great death toll began in our case in the month of January and lasted for the space of seven months. It was of two kinds: the first lasted two months, with continuous fever and spitting of blood, and death occurred within three days. The second lasted for the whole of the remainder of the time, also with continuous fever, and with ulcers and boils in the extremities, principally under the armpits and in the groin, and death took place within five days. And [it] was of so great a contagion (especially when there was spitting of blood) that not only through living in the same house but merely through looking, one person caught it from the other.

De Chauliac instructed the pope to isolate himself entirely and light two large torches as he believed that fire would prevent him from catching the infection. He believed that fire purified the air. Pope Clement was spared the wrath of the plague, and scientists think it was because the heat from the fire prevented infected fleas from ever reaching his body.

Even though the pope's life was no longer in jeopardy, Christian tolerance crumbled throughout Europe. Neighbour turned on neighbour looking for someone to blame. Vicious rumours spread that the Jews were responsible continued to fly, and Catholics retaliated. The Jews were accused of plots to destroy Christendom. The flagellants dragged them from their homes and burned them at the stake in their continued need for a scapegoat. Although Pope Clement condemned these acts, over 5000 Jews were murdered by the time the plague had departed.

The plague of 1348 left as mysteriously as it had come, and while it did make more appearances in the next few hundred years, it would never be as devastating as it was in the fourteenth century. As medical science began to advance, doctors were able to make some headway in recognizing and treating the illness. It wasn't until the late 1800s that Swiss physician and bacteriologist Alexandre Emile Jean Yersin (1863–1943) would identify the bacteria. He was able to understand that the disease had come from infected fleas looking for hosts. And the crowded streets of bustling European cities were the ultimate place to find them. The bacteria responsible for the plague, *Yersinia Pestis*, was named in honour of the man who classified it and shed light on just how it affected people.

The Black Plague indeed was a time where the world was without any hope. People thought God had abandoned them and that judgment day had arrived. From Italy to Ireland, there were millions upon millions left for dead. Millions of people were left in the wake of a disaster that strained every part of European society.

The Black Plague was and remains the worst catastrophe in the history of Europe, but it's also interesting to ponder how the epidemic may have changed history for the better. So many of Europe's cities were overcrowded, filthy, and lacking in morals and structure. With half of their populations gone, there remained a resilience among the people to rebuild. With a smaller population, the people were finally able to get a hold on the filth that had nourished the plague from its beginning.

Urban recovery had become possible with better land suitability and trade. While not all cities would recover at the same rate, many became more productive through the promise of a more industrious world. There was more demand for workers and the peasants who had survived. People were able to ask for better wages and cleaner working conditions. This improved standard of living gave people more power over their lives and would change Europe's future forever.

Chapter Five

A Woman's Duty

Elizabeth of York was known as a kind, dutiful and well-liked queen. Along with her husband, Henry VII, she changed the face of England, and their marriage secured the Tudor dynasty. Elizabeth and Henry were very much in love, and during their seventeen-year marriage, they had many children, but their eighth child, a little girl, survived only about a week, and Elizabeth was to follow. On her birthday, 11 February 1503, Elizabeth of York, Queen of England, lost her life. The king was overcome with grief at the loss of his beloved queen. He locked himself in his chambers, demanding to be left alone in his sadness. He never remarried.

Elizabeth of York is said to have died of childbed fever, an ailment that was unfortunately all too common in medieval Europe. We know today that childbed fever was most likely septicaemia or a uterine infection from lack of a sterile birthing environment. Sadly because of the lack of understanding about the importance of cleanliness and the absence of antiseptic, one in three women died during their childbearing years. While safe from the perils of war, women, however, were not safe from the dangers of pregnancy and childbirth in an archaic and formidable era.

Like almost everything else during the Middle Ages, the Catholic Church was the basis for the thought process for not only life on earth but what came afterwards as well. The entire concept of heaven and hell, sin and good, came from the teachings of the Church. As the Church's beliefs were based on scripture, they saw women as a representation of Eve. Women were a threat to men and full of lustful sin. The Church believed that the consequences of Eve's fall from grace in the book of Genesis were paid for by women as they endured the discomforts of pregnancy. The agony of childbirth, as well as the death or deformity of an infant, only fed the growing distaste the Church felt towards women.

The curse of menstruation was also linked to the sins of Eve. Physicians of the Church taught that menstruation was the body's way of cleansing itself of harmful humours, at least temporarily. Some doctors even called menstruation a sickness. If a woman was afflicted with cramps or a particularly heavy flow, it was assumed that it was God's will. It was believed menstruating women became wicked creatures and their menses only secured the fact that they were far from perfect. Holy women were found not to menstruate, so regular women were viewed as sinners who deserved the distress of menstruation. Some medically minded folks believed that a woman's menses started at her head and travelled through her body, collecting poison and waste from the humours.

Throughout history, women have had to endure not only the ill-conceived notion around their menses but the actual menses themselves, and indeed, the Middle Ages were no different. Hygiene was already a challenge for anyone living during the medieval era, and it must have been even more of one for women during their menses. However, menstruating in the Middle Ages was a lot different than it is today. Luckily for them, medieval women had fewer periods. Women reached menopause much earlier, perhaps in their thirties, and few women had what we would deem as a regular monthly course. This was most certainly the case for women on the lower end of the feudal ladder due to the lack of proper nutrition alone. Peasant women also worked incredibly hard and, no doubt had a smaller percentage of body fat than we do today. The same could be assumed for extremely pious women who had accepted a stringent diet. With a strict diet and lack of proper nourishment, the body would undoubtedly have interruptions in its cycle. The female hormones of oestrogen and progesterone are essential for the overall health of a woman's body, as well as regulating her cycle. Any intense hard work, such as the work endured by serfs and peasant women, would have reduced the level of these crucial hormones in their bodies. The gruelling day-to-day labours of medieval women or those who led a harsh religious life would have had their hormones altered enough to cause irregular cycles. Both poor nutrition and hard work would have resulted in lower body fat, which in turn would have resulted in a sluggish reproductive system. And solely for the fact that a woman's objective was to produce children meant she was, more often than not, pregnant or nursing a child. But of course, medieval women still had their menses, and like today, they had to find a way to deal with it.

What we today call sanitary napkins or pads were made of extra cloth or rags in the Middle Ages. Women preferred to use cotton as it was more absorbent and wool cloth was probably not very comfortable for such an intimate part of the body. The concept of underwear was not yet heard of, and so medieval women had to come up with some way to keep the cloth in place. Perhaps they fashioned some sort of panty-like garment worn close to the body. Some historians have questioned whether or not the plant, sphagnum cymbifolium, a type of moss, would have been used as an absorbent material for menses. The product certainly was porous and had been used as a type of toilet paper and for dressing battlefield wounds. So it would be easy to understand that medieval women found some way to use the moss to act as an absorbent.

When it comes to what we understand as premenstrual syndrome, there was simply no diagnosis in the Middle Ages. It was said to be a melancholia and again seen as the punishment of God upon the female. Physicians saw no need to offer any remedies, but this didn't mean that they weren't available. More often than not, such resources were provided by other women who were well learned in herbal treatment. Thyme and Leaves of Woodruff were regularly made into teas and given for nausea or stomach pain. But there was little else that women could do during their menses to ease the discomfort.

As I will touch upon further in this chapter, it is implausible to see how the medical community deemed menstruating women as a type of monster. One popular belief was that having intercourse with a menstruating woman would produce a horribly deformed child with the red hair of the devil. Some suggested that even looking at a woman during her cycle would cause a venomous toxin to radiate from her eyes. Menstruating women were not allowed to work alongside men in the field, as the very touch of her could cause crops to wilt.

Interestingly enough, most of what was taught about women's medicine during the Middle Ages was based on the theories of Galen and Hippocrates, stemming from a country where women had more freedom to practice medicine and perhaps weren't viewed as such vile creatures. Greek philosophers believed that because a woman's genitals and organs were on the inside, rather than the outside, she was an impacted, botched version of the ideal man. Hippocrates believed that women were colder and more phlegmatic in their humoral makeup. The reason men were viewed as more perfect than women was because of their excess of heat, and heat is nature's instrument. Roman philosopher Gaius Plinius Secundus (23 CE-79 CE) declared that the menstrual blood of women was toxic:

> Contact with it turns wine sour, crops touched by it became barren, grafts die, seeds in gardens dry up, the fruit of the trees fall off, the bright surface of mirrors in which it is merely reflected is dimmed, the edge of steel and the gleam of ivory are dulled, hives of bees die, even bronze and iron are at once seized by rust, and a horrible smell fills the air; to taste it drives dogs mad and infects their bites with incurable poison.

Ironically, all academic study was done by clerics who were men. These men were celibate and would never father children. Also, ironically, one of the most used texts of the literature of the study of women was the *Trotula*, which was written in part by a woman. The *Trotula of Salerno* refers to a group of three texts written by three different physicians during the eleventh century. Trota served not only as a physician but as a lecturer at the medical school in Salerno, Italy. She paid particular attention to women's health and pregnancy-related issues. Long after her death, medieval doctors relied on her medical references to treat female patients. On the subject of menses, the *Trotula* states:

> Women have purgations from the time of twelve winters to the time of fifty winters, although some women have it longer, especially those with a high complexion who are well-nourished with hot meals and hot drinks and live very much in leisure.

Another medical text frequently referred to was *Secreta Mulierum* or *Secrets of Women*. While the writing is attributed to Albertus Magnus (1200–1280), a German Catholic Bishop, there is a dispute that it may have been written by one of his followers. The text circulated in the later Middle Ages and discussed the male view of females in a scientific nature and from a philosophical perspective. The work covers several chapters that are strictly physical, such as *Formation of the Fetus* and *Signs of Conception*, but also delves deeply into how astrology can affect a woman during her pregnancy. What's particularly interesting about this text is the author's opinion on menstruation and the effect it had on women.

> Women are venomous during the time of their flowers and so very dangerous that they poison beasts with their glance and little children in their cots, sully and stain mirrors, and on some occasions, those men who lie with them in carnal intercourse are made leprous.

In a way, this text certainly provides evidence that women, no matter what century they were born in, have always been seen as folks to treat with great caution during their menstrual cycles.

The *Wellcome Apocalypse*, a medieval manuscript produced in Germany in 1420, drew links between medicine and religion in the Middle Ages. It contained sections on the antichrist and the end of days, along with medicine and the prognosis of disease. Male physicians relied heavily on drawings and images of the pregnant female for reference during their medical careers. One of the pictures that were frequently referenced came from the *Wellcome Apocalypse*. The drawing, *The Disease Woman*, looked at pregnancy as a disability or dysfunction. The image shows an anatomical dissection of a woman, who is entirely naked while squatting, with her chest and abdomen exposed. The uterus is represented by a flask-shaped form, which was a form that was commonly found in the twelfth and thirteenth centuries to portray the womb. Although the image shows no foetus in the womb, it clearly shows that there is no operable path for one to exit the body by way of a vaginal delivery. The image is based on the male's imaginations of the inner workings of a woman, as *The Disease Woman* wasn't a medical treatise but more of a reference sheet.

Throughout the Middle Ages, there remained a great reluctance by medical professionals to treat the intimate problems of a woman, including pregnancy. While the reasons given were to respect her modesty, it may have also come from utter distaste as well. It may have been ignorance, or that doctors just didn't show any interest in treating women, but whatever the reason, this rationing only encouraged the practice of midwifery. In the areas of obstetrics and gynaecology, caregivers were predominantly women.

Most midwives were from the lower class and had no formal education. Not that it was required, as many were illiterate as well. Perhaps it didn't matter, as few books were written on midwifery. Midwives predominantly learned from other midwives and women in the communities and through their own experiences with childbirth. If a young girl expressed the desire to become a midwife, she was expected to be at the birth of her siblings and to observe births attended to by other midwives in the family. Midwives were involved with birthing children from all walks of life, whether it was helping those poorest in the village or being paid to serve royalty. Of course, better payment gave better emphasis on a midwife's reputation. While medical doctors may have had different ideas about women in medicine as a whole, midwives were overall welcomed. Fifteenth century Italian physician Anthonius Guainerius (1412–1445) believed that the concept of females in obstetrics was important. He found that women may have been able to diagnose and cure female problems that men just weren't accustomed to understanding. Soranus of Ephesus, the Greek physician who lived during the first or second centuries CE, wrote text that demanded great respect well into the Middle Ages. He insisted that the midwife be:

> literate, with her wits about her, possessed by a good memory, loving work, respectable and generally not unduly handicapped as regard, her senses, sound of limbs, robust and endowed with long, slim fingers and short nails.

Because midwifery was excluded from most early institutions, women turned to natural remedies to help advance their knowledge of how to help their patients best. For the most part, they were respectable and trustworthy, but it is worth mentioning that it sometimes led to false charges of witchcraft. Many women healers were older, and many men were afraid of them and didn't trust them because they simply didn't understand them. Because their limited formal training made them dependent on herbal remedies, there was always the chance that they could be accused of witchcraft. But for the most part, the widespread belief that midwives were associated with the supernatural is unfounded. When witchcraft did become associated with a midwife, it was usually because of an unsuccessful delivery or pregnancy that the public caught wind of. Unfortunately, reliance on natural medicine and a lack of training often brought about both. And if a midwife had several unsuccessful births on her record, which of course were probably not her fault, there was a chance she could be indicted of supernatural interference.

Today, women have the advantage of knowing if they are pregnant as soon as two weeks after conception. A straightforward blood or urine test can provide results with almost 100% accuracy. Women in the Middle Ages weren't so lucky. Most didn't even know they were pregnant until around five months into gestation, when they would experience the "quickening" or movement of the child. If a woman had missed several menses and suspected she was pregnant, then feeling her baby move was a sure enough way to know, along with her growing belly.

Although a woman's duty during the Middle Ages was to procreate, it would be naïve to pretend that there weren't cases in which pregnancy wasn't desired. Because of the Church's influence over women, the idea of birth control was condemned and looked at no different than terminating a pregnancy. A woman who was facing an unwanted pregnancy also had to face the repercussions of the Church. But in cases that can only emulate modern-day situations, such as rape or sex outside of wedlock or worse, medieval women did resort to ending their pregnancies in some instances of desperation. This was not only socially unacceptable but dangerous as well. It was undoubtedly considered a crime to end one's pregnancy willingly, but there remains very little, if any, written on cases of a woman being punished because of it. It would have been immeasurably challenging to find any evidence that a woman had ended her pregnancy. Because a woman's body was a private affair, especially to male doctors, any remains of a pregnancy would have been quickly disposed of.

Practices used to terminate a pregnancy were not only dangerous, but they also weren't overly effective. There are medical texts that note the power of certain herbs and plants in ending a pregnancy. Islamic practitioners had a generous amount of information regarding the use of herbs, and this information slowly made its way into Western culture. There are twelfth-century texts that describe mugwort in great length as a "menstrual tonic" and later writings that discuss its use in expelling foetal tissue after a miscarriage. It would be wise to consider that the herb had been used by women to end an unwanted pregnancy in a time when it was improper to do so. Pennyroyal and juniper are mentioned in several European writings. In one case, in 1574, a cleric from Essex procured a form of juniper for a woman he had gotten pregnant. Other substances mentioned in medieval texts are opium, watercress, and pomegranates. But these writings were being circulated with little to no advice on how these remedies should even be used. In even small amounts, consuming pennyroyal can be toxic. Using opium in the wrong dosage as an abortifacient could not only end the life of the foetus but the woman as well.

Even in a time dominated by religion, there was no shortage of people who were having sex outside of marriage. Adultery was not that uncommon, and there were prostitutes readily available in most medieval cities. The use of contraceptives and drugs to induce an abortion would have been obtainable for the right price. There were other cases where a pregnancy may have been concealed to the best ability of the mother. The ultimate outcome would have been for her to give birth in secret, usually with the help of another woman. So much of what we know about this unfortunate part of pregnancy has not been documented at length. Women in dire straits would have had to turn to each other for help in either ending the pregnancy or birthing the child in secret. A child may have been sent to a monastery for caretaking or left for dead. The Middle Ages were a very threatening time, both for wanted and unwanted children. History is full of stories of "royal bastards", which are illegitimate children born to kings who strayed from the marriage bed. Henry I of England is said to have had over twenty illegitimate children.

But for the most part, especially for a reigning queen, finding out you were pregnant and having a child was something a woman looked forward to. It was every mother's instinct to protect her unborn baby, but in the Middle Ages, without understanding how or why the unborn were put at continuous risk. Aside from the everyday dangers of disease and unsanitary living, there were certain daily habits that medieval women took for granted.

Considering that the drink of choice among most was wine or ale, this most certainly increased the risk of problems during pregnancy. There was very little understanding of how the womb and development of a foetus came about, so it is wise to assume that there was absolutely no reason to think that drinking alcohol could harm one's baby. We know today that because alcohol passes through a mother's blood to her unborn baby, this can cause a plethora of problems. There is a higher risk for miscarriage or stillbirth, and if a child does survive, the consumption of alcohol by the mother increases the risk of lifelong disabilities. Physical abnormalities, learning disabilities, problems with vision or with hearing, as well as the heart, kidney, or bones could have been more easily understood if there had been any written text on

Foetal Alcohol Syndrome Disorder. But as we know, these discoveries were hundreds of years away.

In addition to alcohol, several foods that were more likely to be contaminated with bacteria were also a risk. Uncooked cheeses, eggs, or any undercooked meat or fish could pose a considerable threat to a pregnant mother and her baby by way of listeriosis or salmonella. It wasn't only the food and drink that could put your baby at risk but the vessels they came in as well. Wealthy women, especially, put themselves at risk by using elaborate goblets and plates that were often glazed using lead. The lead would be ingested when they ate or drank, slowly doing damage to them and their babies. Risks to the baby included miscarriage, prematurity, and developmental delays.

Other than walking or being carried in a litter, the only other means of transportation during the Middle Ages was on horseback. This simple pleasure, whether it be during a hunt or going about your chores, posed another risk to an unborn baby. While a mother's womb provides a safe haven to a baby with its cushioning of amniotic fluid, it isn't accident-proof. Because most women didn't even know they were pregnant until late into the second trimester, riding horseback was especially risky. There is little to protect a baby from harm if one were to get thrown from a distressed horse, or possibly worse, being kicked by one. Not to mention the jostling motion of horseback riding itself can increase the risk of placental abruption, which, unfortunately in the Middle Ages, would most likely mean the death of both the mother and her baby.

A woman of noble birth who had the luxury of a personal physician might have been given what would be known as a very primitive urinalysis. If her urine was whitish or pale and cloudy, the assumption was that a woman might be pregnant—a needle left in the urine to see if it rusted indicated pregnancy. And by the sixteenth century, physicians were able to understand that mixing urine with wine was another way to determine if a woman was with child, as the alcohol in the wine reacted with the proteins in the urine of pregnant women. However, the only 100% foolproof way to determine whether one was going to be a mother was the actual birth itself.

There was no other time that this would prove to be true than in the false pregnancy of Queen Mary I (1516–1558). On 9 July 1553, Mary Tudor was declared Queen of England, and she knew her number one duty was to produce an heir to keep her Protestant sister Elizabeth off the throne. The following July 1554, Queen Mary married King Philip II of Spain (1527–1598). She was thirty-eight years old, and although she understood she was at the end of her childbearing years, she was confident that God would bring her an heir.

By September of that same year, Mary believed she was pregnant and said she felt her baby move in her womb by the end of that month. Her doctors didn't know the difference between a legitimate pregnancy and a false one, and so they took her at her word. With her father-in-law, Charles V of Spain, delighted at the news, Mary now had the future of England and Spain in her womb. By late autumn, it was affirmed that the queen's belly was growing and that her gowns no longer fit. Preparations for her confinement began in April 1555, as her doctors estimated that she would deliver in May. But there was something different about the queen, and her doctors were worried about her mental state. She seemed almost depressed, unstable, and had stopped eating. Doctors were growing more concerned about the nutrition of the baby.

April and May came and went with rumours of a birth, but by June and July, there was no baby. The queen insisted her timing was off and that the baby was definitely coming. But the people began to pity her behind her back for her delusions. During the month of August, 11 months into her "pregnancy", Mary came out of her confinement thin, silent, and humiliated. Whether it was cancer or a tumour that had caused the growth in Mary's stomach, we will never know. But the word pregnancy was never mentioned again in her court.

Because of the strong influence of the Catholic Church, besides Eve, there was another woman who played an essential role in the lives of pregnant women. The ultimate mother, the Virgin Mary. Mary was the epitome of the maternal caretaker. She was the mother of Jesus Christ, and this made her the perfect mother, the nurturer. And one that women in the Middle Ages looked to for their strength. The Church was consistent in showing Mary as a role model. She was always presented as a chaste, perfect woman who was constantly praying. Fifteenth century art especially depicted Mary in such a way. She was eloquent like a courtly lady, who displayed knowledge and divinity like a heavenly queen. The Virgin Mary was looked at as the intercessor; she was the connection to God and Heaven. She was called on for protection in an unstable world by pregnant and birthing mothers. Women went to great lengths to pay homage to both Mary and other saintly women, whom they believed could offer assistance. Pilgrimages were considered the most direct route to ask for the intercession of a saint.

In 1061, the village of Walsingham in Norfolk, England, became associated with repeated Marian apparitions, and a shrine was erected in her name. It soon became a place of pilgrimage. In 1453, Margaret of Anjou (1430–1482), queen to King Henry VI (1421–1471), travelled to Our Lady of Walsingham in desperation for a child. She offered a richly, bejewelled golden tablet as a gift, the most expensive thing she owned. The offering also showed the importance of fertility. Her trip was noted in a letter from Cecily Neville, Duchess of York (1414–1495):

> It pleased thereunto in your coming from that blessed, gracious and devout pilgrimage of Our Lady of Walsingham to suffer the coming of my simple person.

Her pilgrimage paid off. Just a few months later, Margaret of Anjou became pregnant. Countless other men and women made the pilgrimage to Our Lady of Walsingham to ask the Virgin Mary to pray for them. And because Mary is particularly associated with matriarchal duties, women especially travelled to the shrine to ask for her blessing. Queen Katherine of Aragon (1485–1536), a devout Catholic, was a regular pilgrim to the shrine. Katherine suffered several miscarriages throughout her marriage, and her faith and comfort in the Holy Mother would remain a consistent part of her life.

Katherine of Aragon also visited Frideswide Shrine in Oxford. In April 1518, the queen was on route with the court when she stopped to visit the shrine. Already pregnant, Katherine prayed in desperation for a healthy male heir. Sadly her prayers went unanswered as she delivered a stillborn daughter in November later that year. Frideswide Shrine is named after a Saxon Princess and healer, who later became the Patron Saint of Oxford. Believed to be from the 700s, she was a young woman, who having vowed herself to Christ, became a nun. She was pursued relentlessly by the King of Leicester for her hand in marriage. She fled in desperation, begging for God's protection. God struck the king blind a so he asked for Princess Frideswide's forgiveness. She granted it, and the king's sight was restored.

She has since been remembered as a figure of virtue and one who can offer great healing.

The Shrine of St. Thomas Becket (1119–1170) at Canterbury Cathedral was a place of great pilgrimage since being built in 1220. It had been a place where people travelled to ask for blessings for themselves, sick family members, and their farm animals. Becket became Archbishop of Canterbury in 1162 but was murdered in his own cathedral in 1170. He was given sainthood by the Catholic Church soon after his death. Becket was known for his connections with fertility and childbirth and has been venerated for helping infertile women. Many of Becket's miracles were recounted by William of Canterbury, an English monk and biographer of the saint's wonders. One such tale tells of a time that Saint Becket intervened to save both the mother and baby during a complicated breech birth. According to a parish priest, who had been there with them at the shrine, the only solution was to amputate the baby's trapped arm as it had been "swollen to the thickness of a man's leg". The mother then drank the water from Becket's shrine, and "the hand was withdrawn, and the foetus turned and presented normally through the intervention of St. Thomas".

The wife of Henry III, Eleanor of Provence, visited the shrine for assistance with her pregnancy in 1244. She gave thanks by presenting one thousand half-pound candles to the shrine. A stained-glass window from Canterbury Cathedral shows a woman offering candles, such as those that had been used at Becket's tomb by a woman who nearly died of childbirth. The woman was cured after her husband offered a large candle the length of his wife to the tomb. Margaret of Anjou also made several visits there. Early in her reign, she went in September 1446 to hear Mass at the shrine, and the following September, she made the pilgrimage to Canterbury on foot. She much desired a pregnancy and asked time and again for the assistance of Saint Becket.

The protection of the Virgin Mary was also asked for in the form of birth girdles. Birth girdles, or prayer rolls, were a lengthy piece of parchment placed over the belly of an expectant or birthing mother. The girdles were inscribed with blessings and prayers and promised a safe delivery of the child. The girdles said to be in proportion to the height of the Virgin Mary also showed various scenes of the crucifixion of Christ. Girdles were used by mothers to call upon saints during long and complicated labours. Words that were written or spoken may have been words that were said by Christ himself. Texts also included depictions of Mary's painless delivery in the hopes that labouring women may find strength during their ordeal. For women, these prayer rolls offered protection from the two most significant dangers of childbirth, the death of the mother and the death of the child itself. Along with wearing a birth girdle, the woman and those surrounding her would immerse themselves in intercessory prayer and meditation over the wounds of Christ. In 1502, great rewards were given to a monk for delivering "our Lady gyrdelle" to Queen Elizabeth of York six weeks before giving birth to her eleventh child.

Labouring and pregnant women also prayed to St. Margaret of Antioch, who lived during the third century and was tortured and then executed because of her Christian faith. St. Margaret is linked to women in labour because while in prison, she was supposedly visited by Satan, who was disguised as a dragon. After his attempts to swallow her whole, the cross she carried caused him to spit her back out. Because she came out of the dragon unscathed, pregnant women looked to her in prayer that their own babies were born healthy.

While we understand that several pregnant or soon to be pregnant women went to great lengths to visit shrines of their beloved saints, there seem to be few miracles concerning childbirth in hagiographical literature. These beautiful works of art tell us such a remarkable story. We can reflect on the many wonders that are connected with a saint's tomb or shrine. Written in the year 1260, *The Golden Legend* is a compilation of hagiographies that was popular in the later Middle Ages. It was written by Jacobus de Varagine (1230–1290), an Italian chronicler from the city of Genoa. And yet, we have little to go on when it comes to the lives of pregnant women. Historians who study the lives of saints in depth can help us to understand why.

Before the late twelfth century, one was expected to make the pilgrimage to the shrine and be in physical contact with it before expecting a miracle. People often dropped to their knees after miles of travel or laid down at the foot of the church to sleep for the night. But women who may have been in the pangs of extended labour couldn't be expected to make such a journey. If a mother were in the throes of a difficult birth, she would be in no condition to travel and probably would have been forbidden it by her husband anyway. And so, the idea of appealing to a saint from your birthing bed began to take hold. Instead of further risking the lives of the mother and child, it became more common for folks to call for a saint from the safety of their home. This gives us an idea of why there weren't public records of an expecting mother's journey to a shrine because it was probably pretty rare. But it doesn't mean that there weren't any stories of a pregnant woman's quest for a miracle. There remain texts from earlier in the twelfth century that indicate pregnant women did make the journey to a shrine seeking help. Perhaps their stories were shared with monastic superiors at the shrines and maybe not written up into proper form. An early twelfth century reference to women visiting the shrines of saints was found in the *Vita Sancti Benigni*, written by William of Malmesbury (1095–1143). William was an English historian and monk who wrote extensively on logic and physics. He refers to the miracles of St. Benignus (d 467) regarding pregnancy, writing about "women who carried dead foetuses in their wombs".

While it is difficult to interpret what miracles may have befallen women with foetal demise, his writings confirm that women did go to the shrine of St. Benignus for help with their pregnancies.

History's medieval women who stood at the middle and bottom of the feudal system didn't leave us with many written accounts of their pregnancies, but there were those who did; royals. Mainly because women of the lower class either weren't educated enough or simply because nobody felt it was important to document such events in people who weren't of noble stature. But the lives of royal women were relevant and well documented.

The birth of a monarch was a substantial political event for all to witness, not a private affair. The pressure placed on a pregnant queen to deliver a son was tremendous, so much so that it was unfathomable even to think that the baby could be a female. A sizeable healthy family was a symbol of strength to the entire nation. The reign of the Plantagenets, beginning with Henry II in 1154 and ending with Richard III in 1485, spanned over 330 years. The dynasty proved a strong bloodline with fourteen ruling kings of England. Queens knew their duty to the realm and knew that their position greatly depended on birthing a healthy son. A queen's success was defined by whether or not she could produce a healthy male heir for the kingdom. If there was the failure of a son to arrive, the blame was put on the queen. A queen who could not bear children was proof that God looked unfavourably upon the kingdom. The entire reign of Henry VIII was based on whether or not he had a male heir. His first two wives had been completely marginalised for their failure to give him a son. His first wife, Katherine of Aragon, had countless miscarriages, and Henry's disappointment in her caused their divorce. And when his second wife, Anne Boleyn, delivered a premature son, who may have been malformed, she was to blame. The king believed that God looked down upon his marriages and showed his displeasure by denying him a male heir.

Several weeks to a month or so before the expected delivery of an heir, preparations for a queen's lying-in would start. The lying-n was the time that a queen would disappear from courtly life as she prepared for her baby. The queen was usually tucked away in her chambers, with only a few of her ladies to tend to her. All the windows in the queen's chambers were shut tight and covered with thick tapestries, as no fresh air was allowed in the room. These tapestries were covered with serene religious scenes or picturesque landscapes. Too much light was considered dangerous, and so very little, if any, was allowed in the room. The idea behind all of this was to recreate the safety and calmness of the womb. Fires would be lit, even in summer, and the Queen's ladies were instructed to only speak in a whisper. Anything too loud or too bright could upset her or her baby. Without any fresh air, there was little hope for a pleasant smell, but attempts were made with herbs and rushes placed about the floor. These rushes were replaced more often than as if they had been laid anywhere else.

Once a queen had safely delivered an heir, she still needed to be hidden from the public until she could be reintroduced to society. Although her baby would have been immediately christened, she would not have attended the event. She was considered unclean because of her condition, both physically and mentally. She had, after all, as the Church believed, endured the sin of Eve, royal or not. A queen had to be churched, or blessed, by a priest, six weeks after the birth of her baby.

But even a queen was not immune to the horrors of childbirth and the dangers that followed. In a time when people would never know the blessings of a sterile hospital room or the promise of antibiotics to save the life of your baby, women suffered tremendously through the perils of childbirth.

Because men dominated the world of education, texts adhering to pregnancy were rare, and midwives had to rely on their instinct, as well as what limited resources they had. And these resources were written by men who hadn't a strong understanding of how the female reproduction system worked. Apart from the teachings of Hippocrates and Galen, the few texts available during the Middle Ages were more of a shot in the dark than an accurate description of medical procedures or cures.

Perhaps the most heard of text available to midwives was that of Soranus of Ephesus. His writings seemed to have the most accurate observations on the nature of the uterus. Soranus seemed to understand that pregnancy came in stages, and one of the most critical was the first three months. But the knowledge of this crucial time would have proved almost useless, as it was rare that most women understood that they were with child that early in the pregnancy. Soranus also wrote on the expected birthing positions of a foetus and how a midwife may have to turn the child manually. He encouraged hot baths, poultices, and applications of herbs to ease labour. So, while his texts were written during the first century CE, the sensibilities of his writing proved a stronghold throughout time and became an invaluable tool to midwives and physicians during the Middle Ages.

Another series of texts that played a role in obstetrics during the Middle Ages was the Sloane Manuscripts. These manuscripts are a collection of medical documents that were put together in the eighteenth century by physician Sir Hans Sloane (1660–1753). These texts hold copies of the writings of a fourteenth century Italian physician, Roger Frugardi (1140–1195), called *Practica Chirurgiae* (The Practice of Surgery). They also hold copies of Henry VIII's medical recipes and a fifteenth century physician's almanac. These texts also played a vital role in the education and reference to female medicine, along with chemistry, botany, magic, and religion.

It goes without saying that enduring the pain of childbirth without anaesthetic must have been excruciating. Millions of brave women still experience this pain today, but they do so in an environment where trained midwives or physicians closely monitor them. The risk of complications remains small in comparison to the Middle Ages, and women now have the security of knowing that medical intervention is at their fingertips. Women in the Middle Ages were offered very little to ease their physical discomfort. While holy relics and amulets may have provided some solace, they likely did little to ease the burden of pain. And these would have to have been things the Church was okay with. As long as it came from natural properties, it was assumed that it came from God. A mother may have been given a sip of wine or a herbal remedy for strength. A drink called a *caudle* made up of eggs, cream, porridge, and ale may have warmed her belly, but that was it. And physical discomfort was the least of one's worries. Childbirth was dangerous, and there was no getting around it. There was no way to monitor the mother throughout the pregnancy, or the birth and conditions like eclampsia would have surely meant the untimely demise of one or both. The loss of a mother or the baby was always feared. In 1533, Queen Anne Boleyn wrote her will before her lying-in during her pregnancy with her first child. It was common for women to do so, and the loss of a queen would have been unimaginable.

History is filled with tragic stories of queens who died in childbirth. Queen Isabella of Hainault (1170–1190), wife of King Philip II of France (1165–1223), died while giving birth to twins. Isabella was only ten years old when she married fourteen-year-old Philip. Under French law, Isabella was not yet of age for the consummation of the marriage. But by 1183, when Philip was crowned King, he was more than ready for an heir. Isabella had gained the favour of the people. Her first son was born healthy in 1187, but it would be another three years before she would become pregnant again. This pregnancy would prove very difficult for her, and on 14 March 1190, she gave birth to twin boys. Sadly, Isabella died only a day later, and her twins followed her to the grave three days after that. Tragically, her life was cut short after complications during the birth. She was not yet twenty years old and had been a popular queen. The people of France mourned her. Isabella of Mar (1277–1296), wife of Scottish king Robert the Bruce, died in childbirth as well. Legend states that the couple was very much in love. Isabella was quick to become pregnant, and although she had a healthy and unremarkable pregnancy, she died after giving birth to a daughter. Isabella was only nineteen years old. Her daughter, who was named Margorie (1296–1316), in honour of the King's mother, also died in childbirth. Sources tell of a riding accident that happened when Margorie was pregnant. She had married Walter Stewart, 6th High Steward of Scotland (1293–1327). On 2 March 1316, Margorie was far along in her pregnancy when her horse was startled, and she was thrown to the ground. She went into premature labour, and her son, the future King Robert II (1316–1390), was born. Like her mother, Margorie was also around age nineteen when she died. The story of her death remains unproven as to whether she died at the birth of her son or shortly after.

In a perfect delivery, a baby would be born in the ideal head down position and come into the world with considerable ease, and all would be well. And while this did happen, there was still a good chance that things could go horribly wrong. When they did, women had to endure the entire ordeal, sometimes quite traumatically. This was the case for Lady Margaret Beaufort, Countess of Richmond. Margaret became a bride at the age of twelve in an arranged marriage to Edmund Tudor (1430–1456). While twelve was considered young even then for a wedding to be consummated, Margaret was considered very valuable, and her new husband wasted no time in getting her pregnant. Her husband died six months later, leaving Margaret, thirteen years old, pregnant, and scared. Margaret was a petite girl, unfit for labour to begin with, and the delivery was said to have been almost enough to kill her. While she did finally give birth to a healthy baby boy, she never conceived again. When Margaret's nine-year-old granddaughter was married to a man ten years her senior, Margaret made her views very clear that the marriage was not to be consummated right away.

Perhaps one of the most common complications of childbirth was when the baby presented in a manner that was not going to ensure a smooth delivery. Although the writings of Trota of Solerno were in great part about women, very little was written on the act of birthing itself. In fact, there was very little text written on delivery at all. In the academic books of Bartholomeus Anglicus (1203–1272), which were popular in the fourteenth and fifteenth centuries, there was only one chapter written on childbirth, and it was quite limited. What was available for reference were the Sloane Manuscripts, along with the writings of a few other Greek physicians. Aetios of Amida (502–575), who had been court doctor to Justinian, Emperor of Byzantium (d 565 AD), had dealt with difficult deliveries and his writings on breech delivery were referred to. He wrote:

> of the remaining positions, that which is less dangerous is a foot
> presentation, particularly if the foetus comes out with a hand

extended over each thigh. The foetus which comes out by one foot while the other foot is retained or those with both feet doubled up and leaning on either side of the vulva need straightening as do those who have outstretched hands.

Arabian physician Rhazes (865–925), whose works were held in high regard in the west, wrote that a head presentation should require no manual interference but that other presentations may require the hand of a midwife to be inserted to help correct the baby. He also advised on anointing the genitals with oil to stimulate labour and ease the baby's transition.

It is clear to us today that by looking at the various illustrations in medieval medical texts, that physicians had no real understanding of the womb or how the foetus grew and developed. Most figures show a man child, or a child, nearing the age of two with masses of hair, floating aimlessly in a "uterus" that was more shaped like a lightbulb. These drawings only solidified the fact that instructions on how to turn a baby were very impractical and would be of no help at all to a midwife trying to help a labouring mother.

The Sloane Manuscripts make several references to difficult birthing positions and ways to ensure a safe delivery. While the right idea may have been there, these attempts frequently led to failure. Anointing the birth canal with hot herbs and oils while trying to coax the cervix to open further would have most likely introduced infection if nothing else. There are recommendations to push the child back up into the womb to keep them warm until a resolution had been decided. If a child wasn't in the correct position for birth, according to the Sloane Manuscripts, it was due to an unnatural sickness in childbearing and could be presented in sixteen different ways. Most of these being challenging positions such as transverse, footlong, footlong breech, etc. All of which today would have been delivered via caesarean section as they quickly resulted in maternal exhaustion or foetal distress. But because surgery wasn't an option unless the mother had passed, other techniques were offered. The Walcher Position is referred to as well, which is a position that encourages the mother to recline with her back and legs dangling, her bottom propped up by several pillows. This position was thought to ease the delivery of a baby that may have needed to be turned before passing through the birth canal. The birthing stool, which can be traced back to 1450 BCE

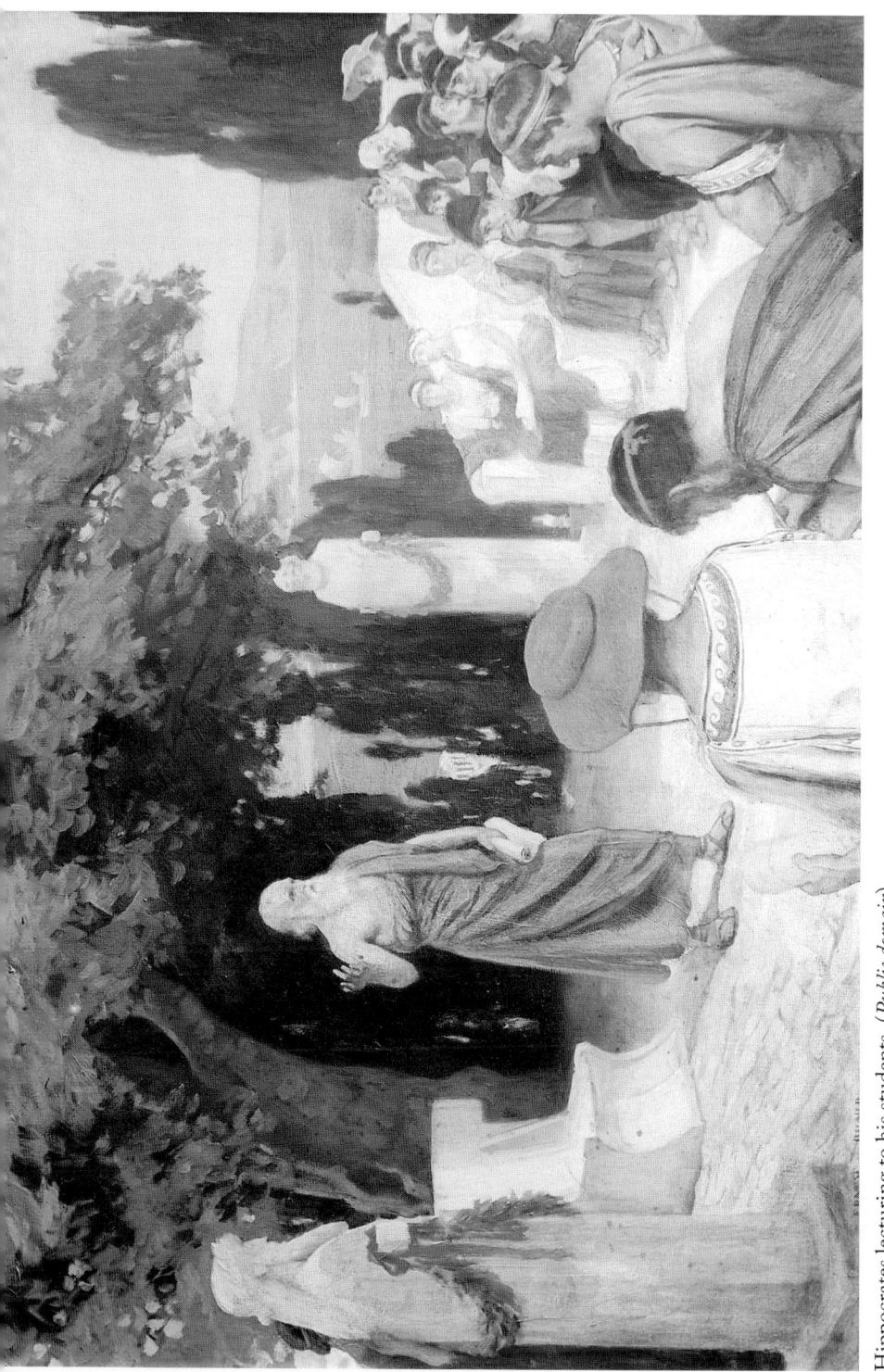

Hippocrates lecturing to his students. (*Public domain*)

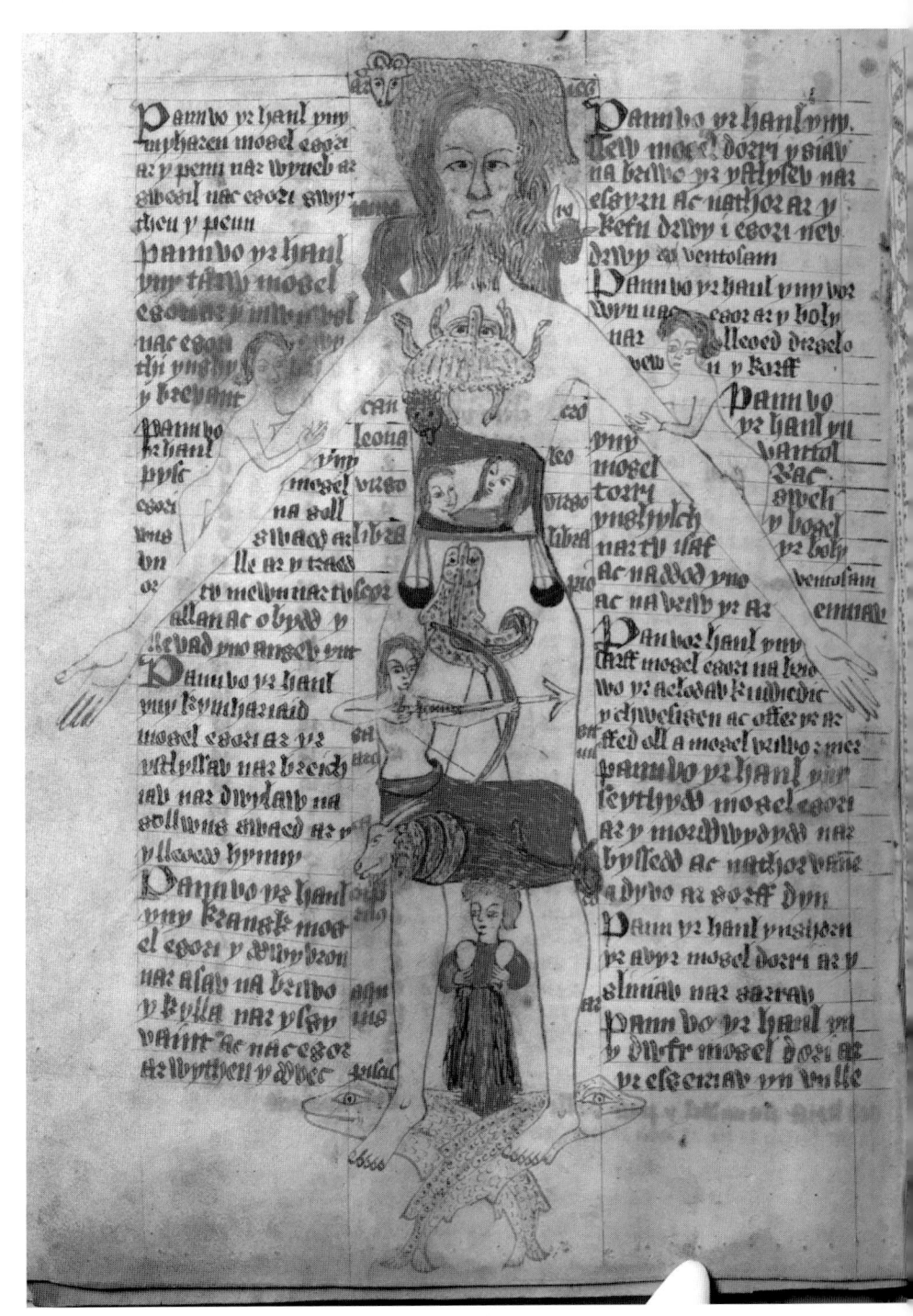

15th century drawing of Zodiac Man. (*Public domain*)

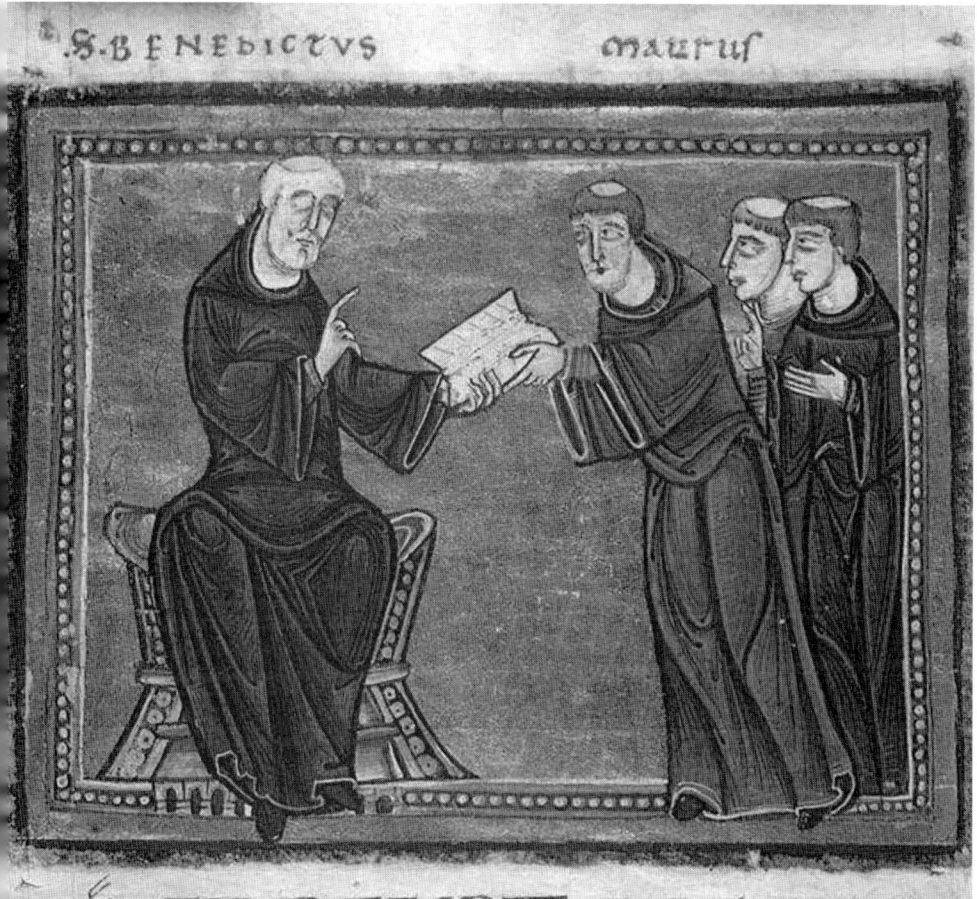

12th century drawing of St. Benedict delivering his Orders. (*Public domain*)

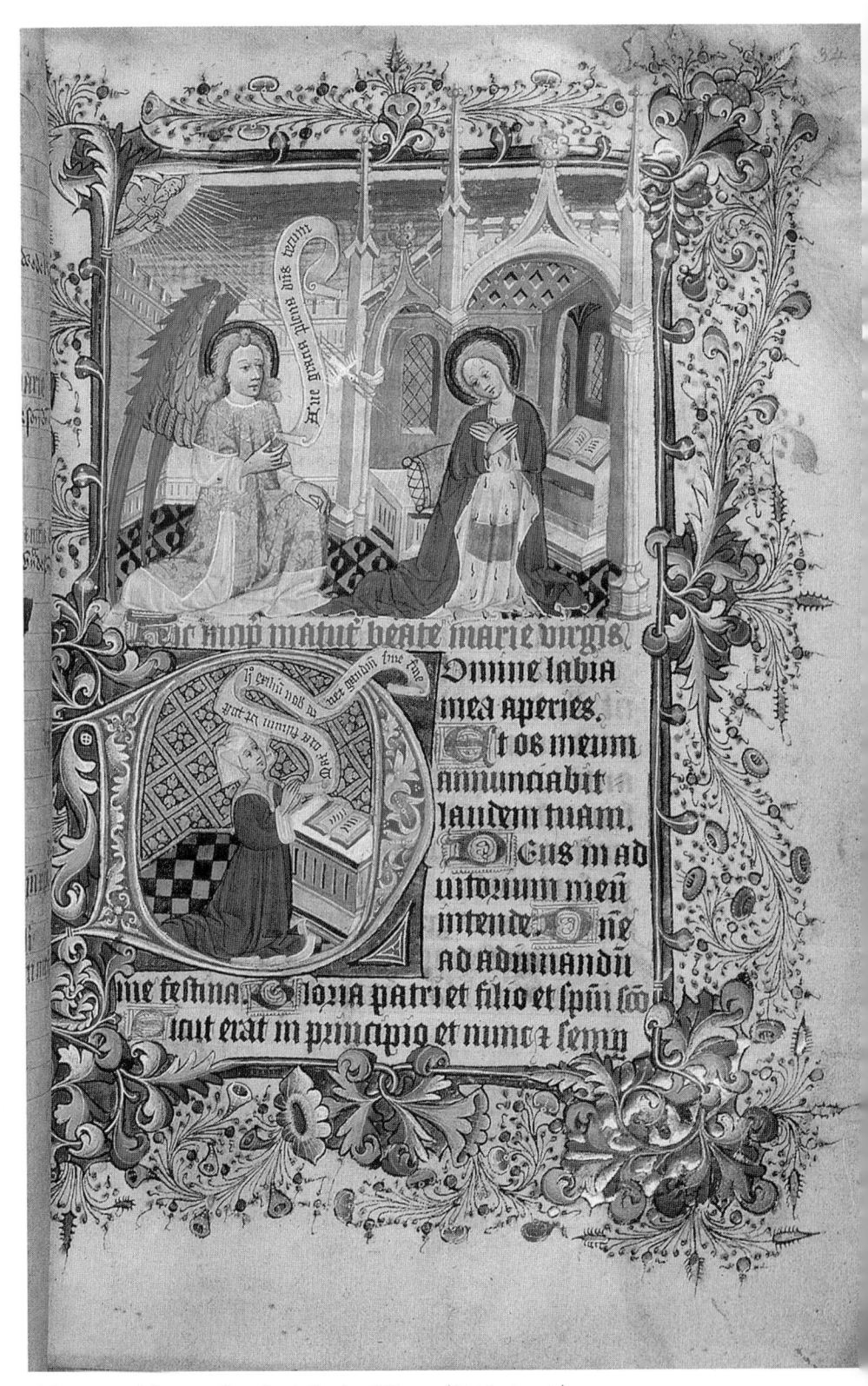

15th century, Margaret Beaufort's Book of Hours. (*Public domain*)

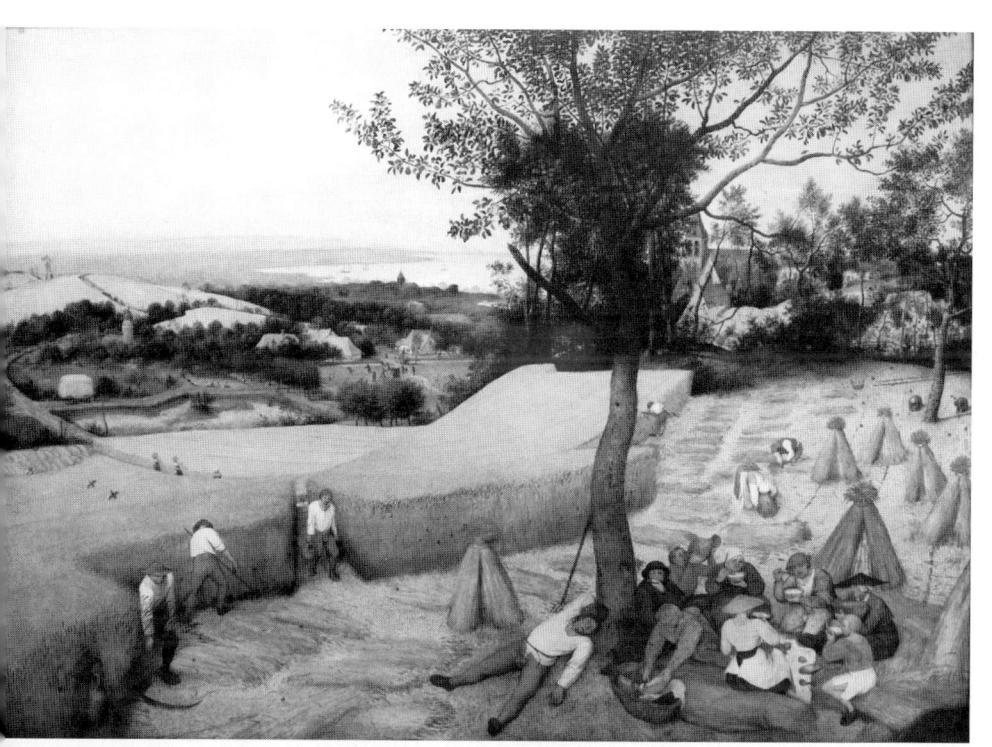

16th century painting by Pieter Bruegel, 'The Corn Harvest'. Life for the medieval serf. (*Public domain*)

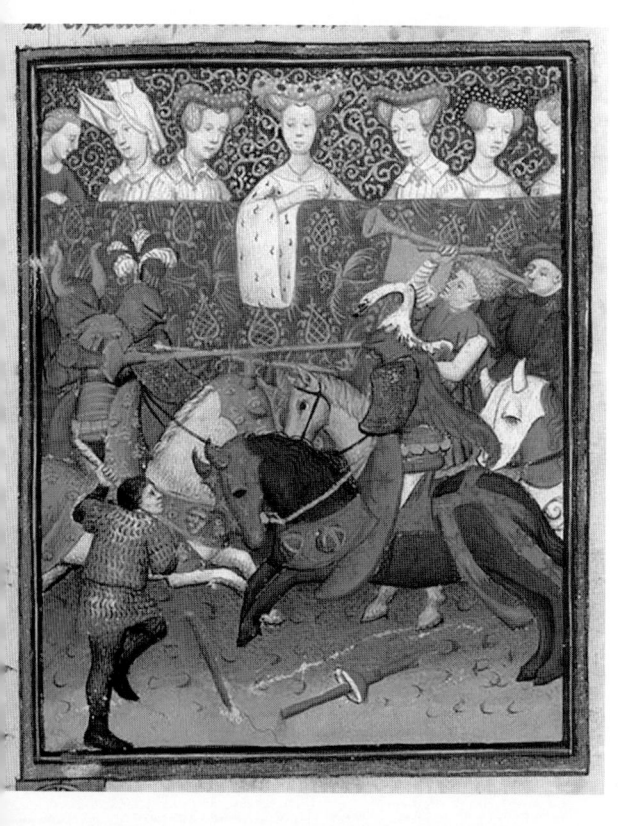

15th century drawing of ladies watching knights joust. (*Public domain*)

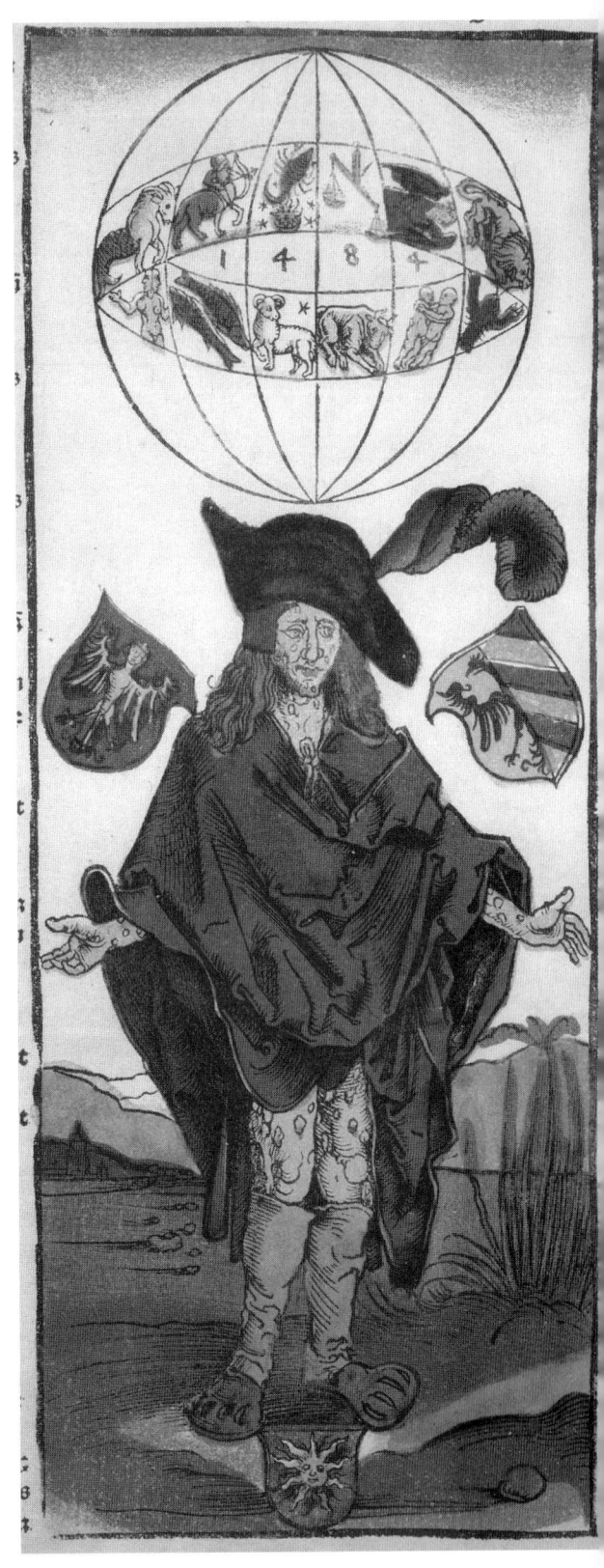

15th century drawing showing details of a syphilitic man. (*Public domain*)

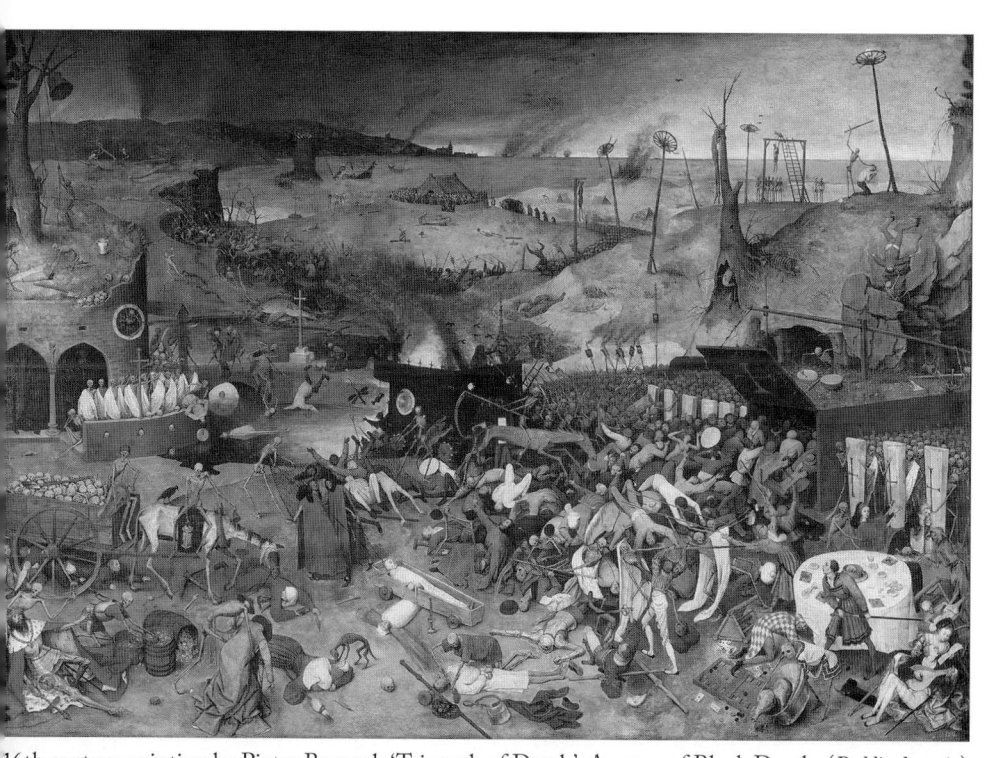

16th century painting by Pieter Bruegel, 'Triumph of Death'. A scene of Black Death. (*Public domain*)

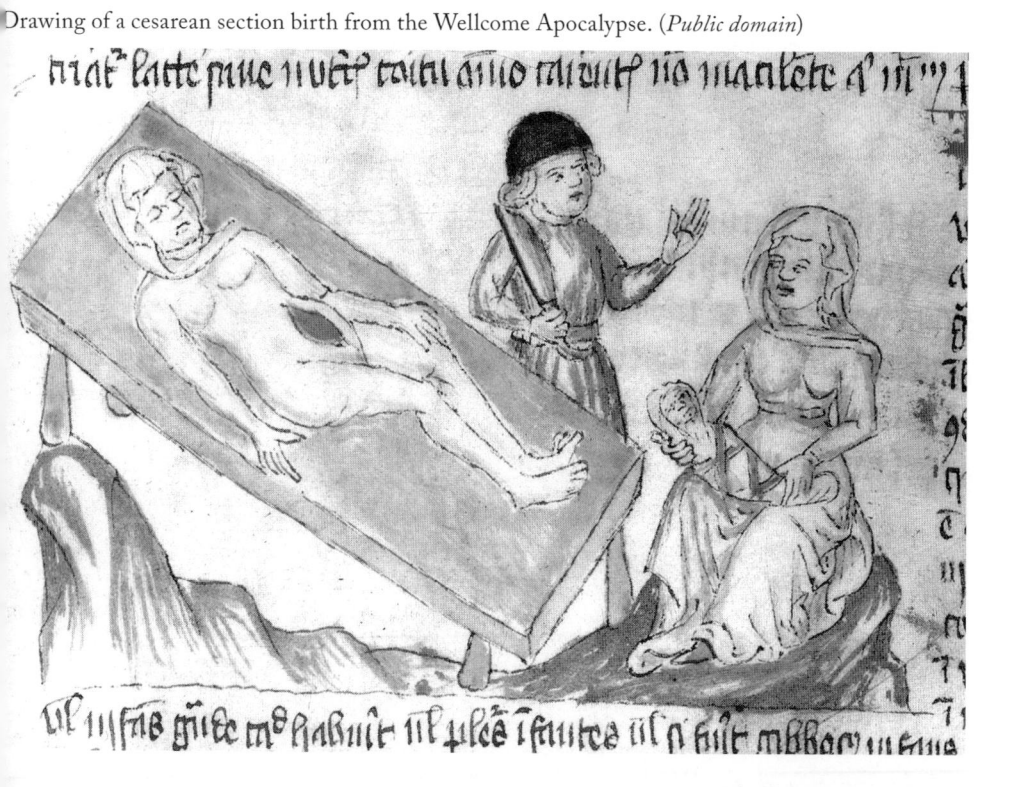

Drawing of a cesarean section birth from the Wellcome Apocalypse. (*Public domain*)

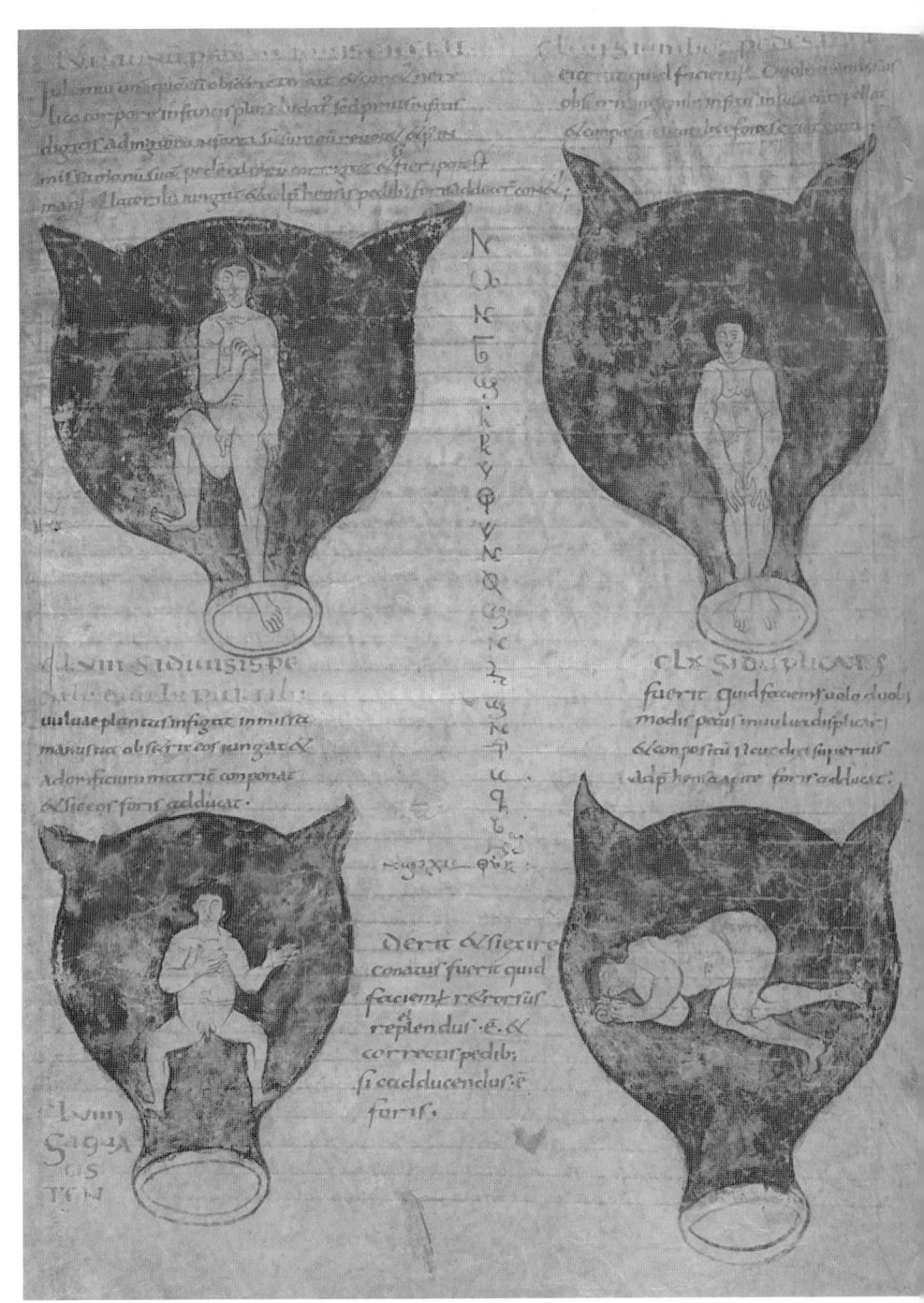

9th century drawing of various fetal positions. (*Public domain*)

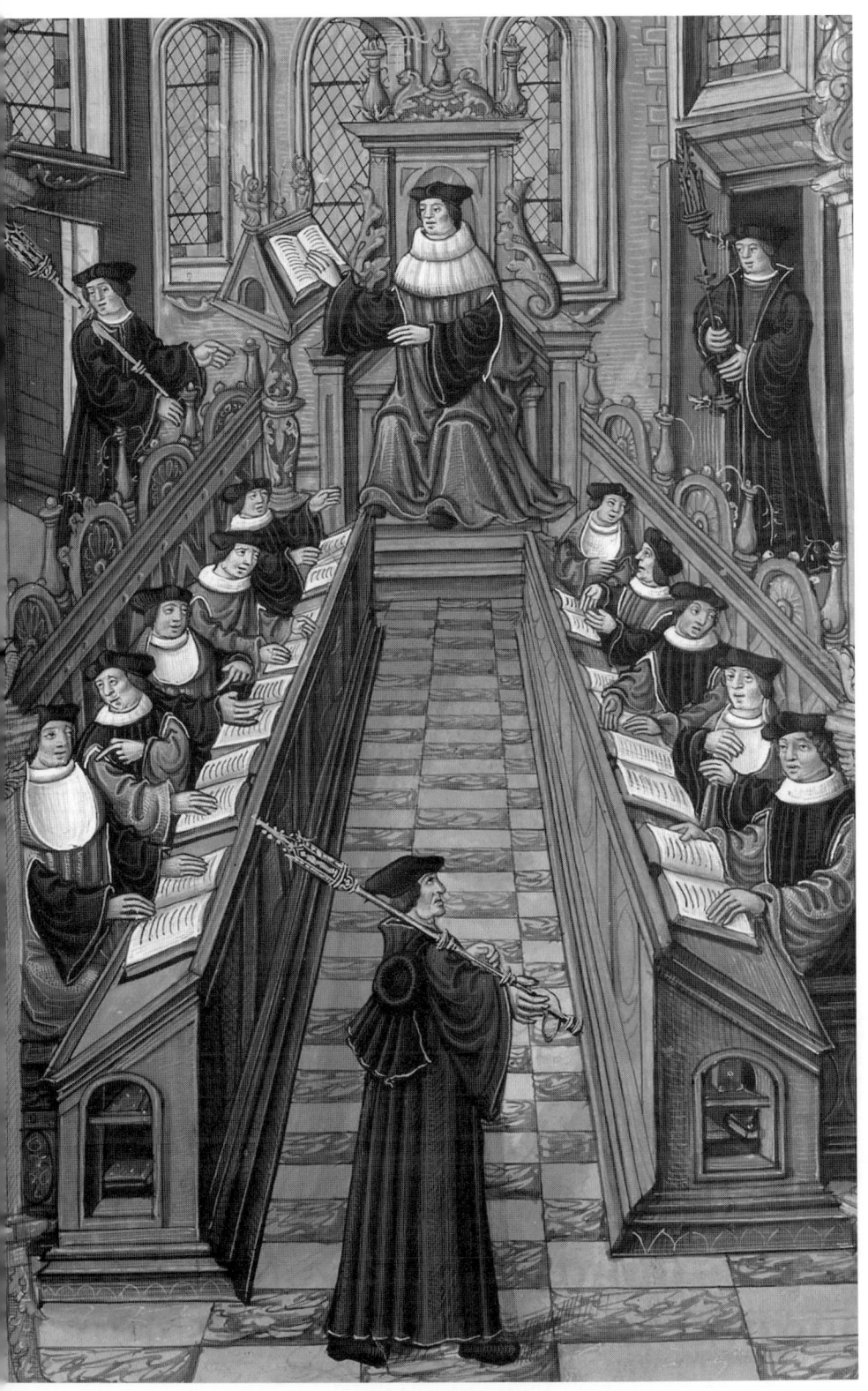

16th century drawing of student doctors at the University of Paris. (*Public domain*)

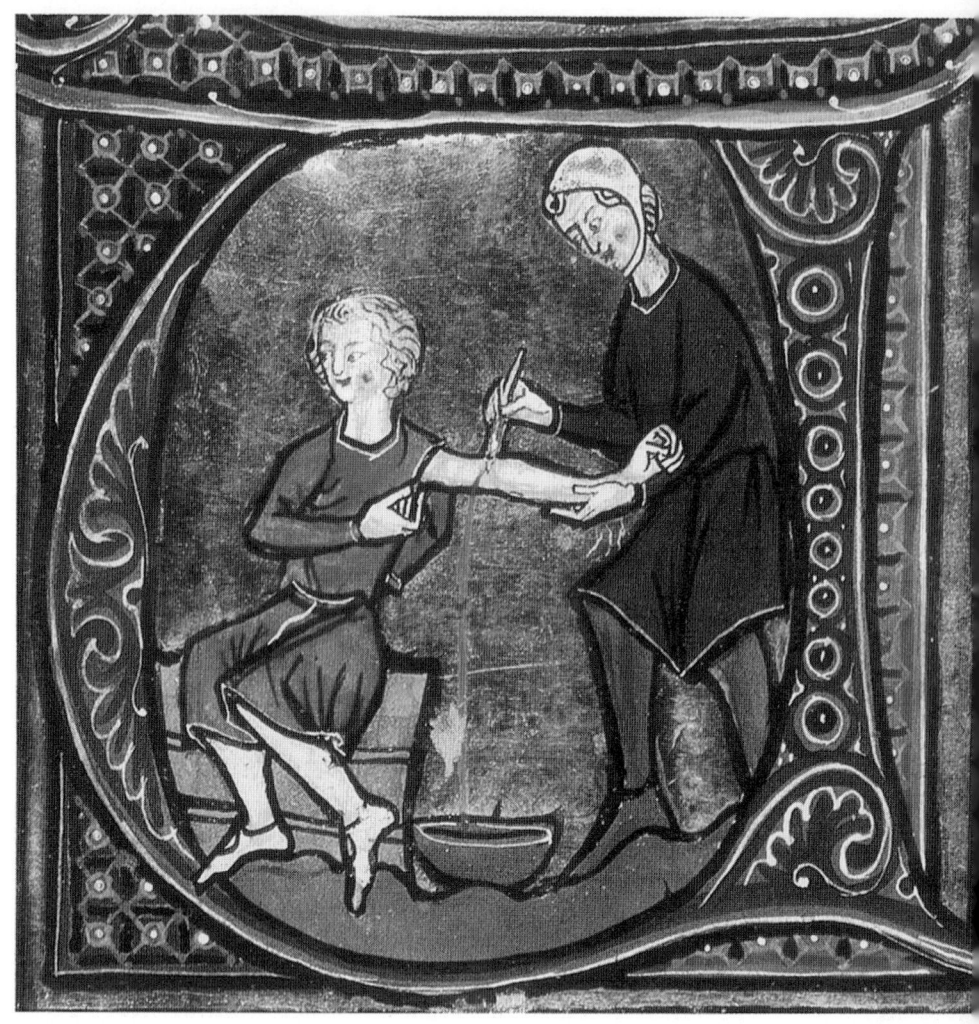

13th century drawing of bloodletting. (*Public domain*)

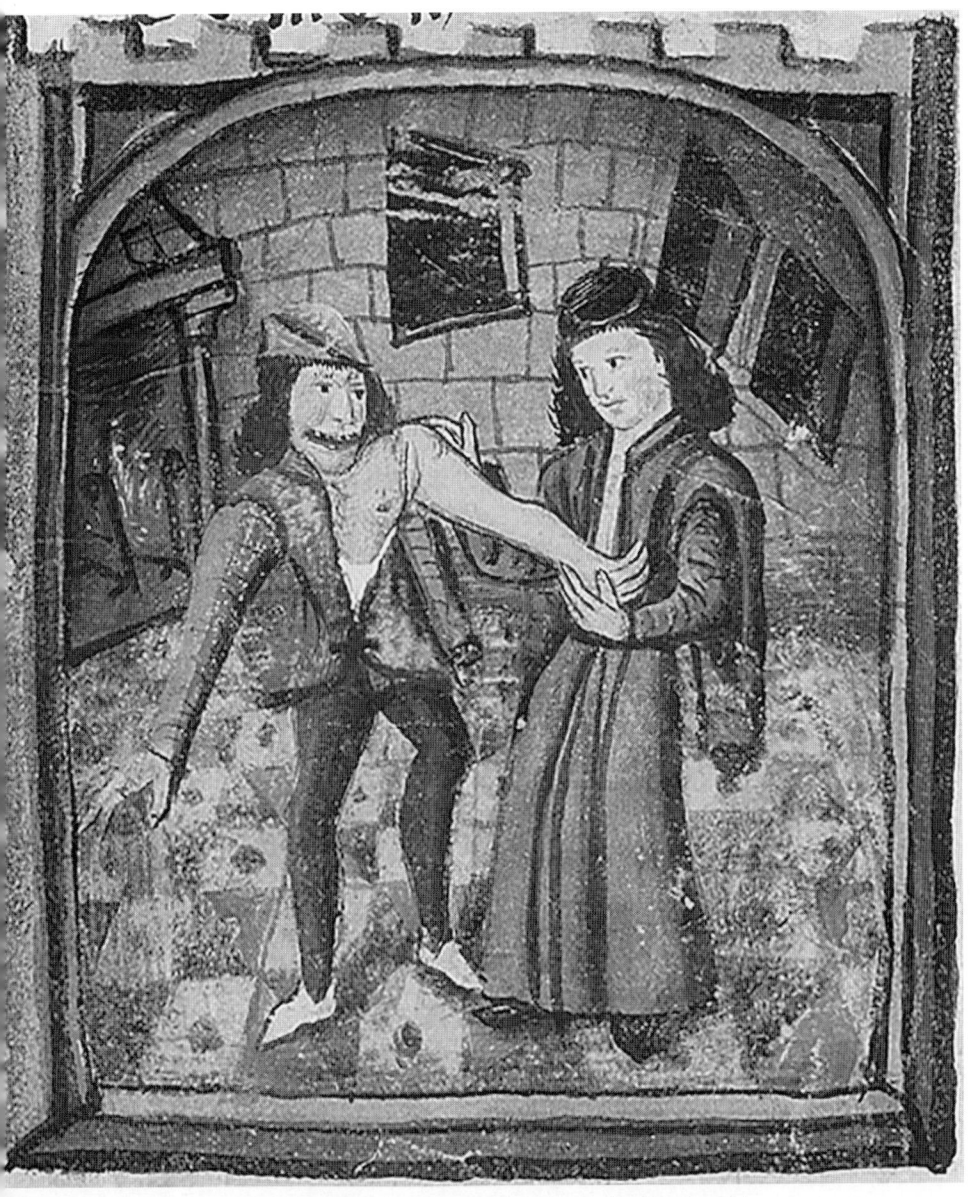

15th century drawing of Guy de Chaulic setting a broken bone. (*Public domain*)

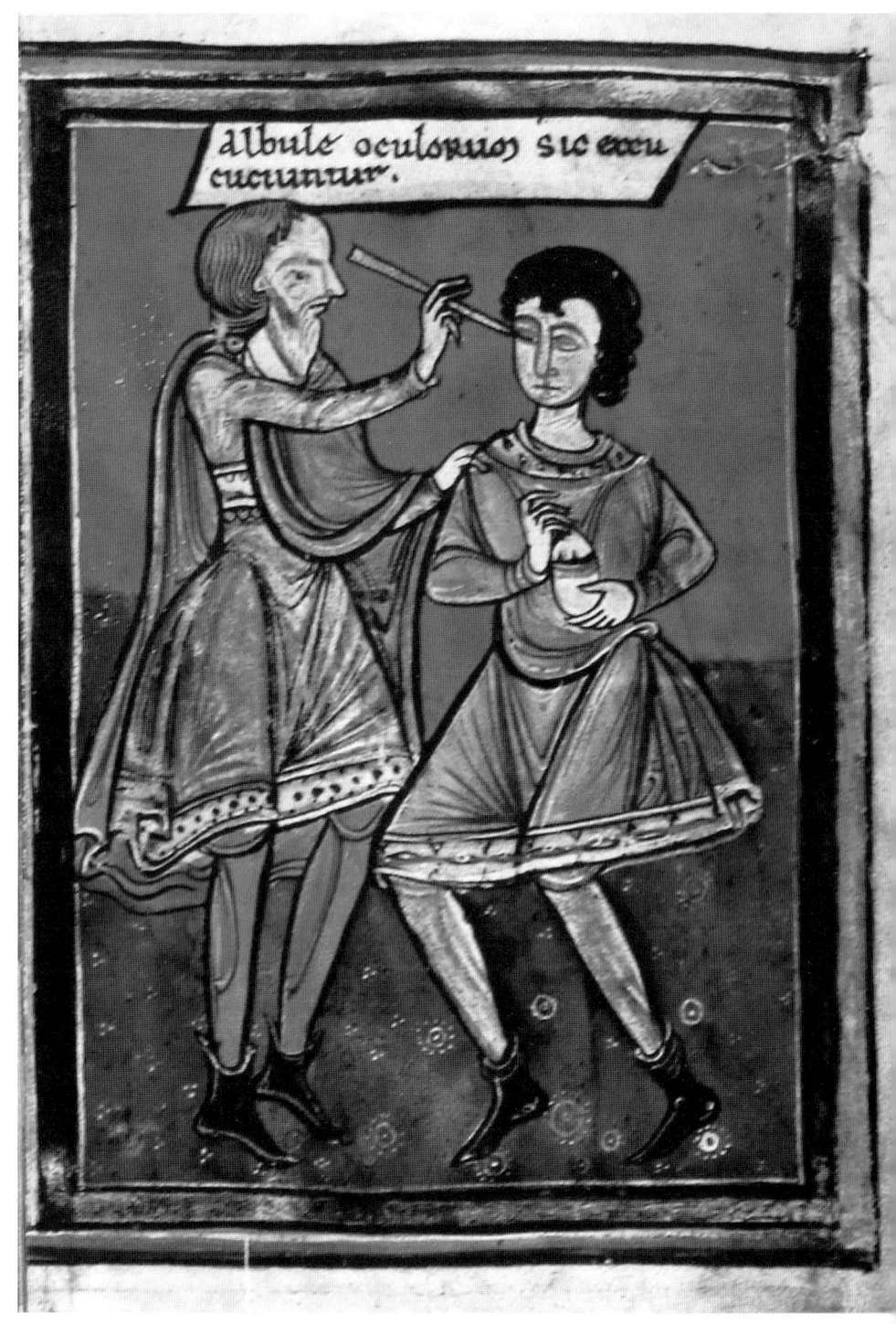

12th century drawing of ocular surgery. (*Public domain*)

1902 drawing of Henry V. (*Public domain*)

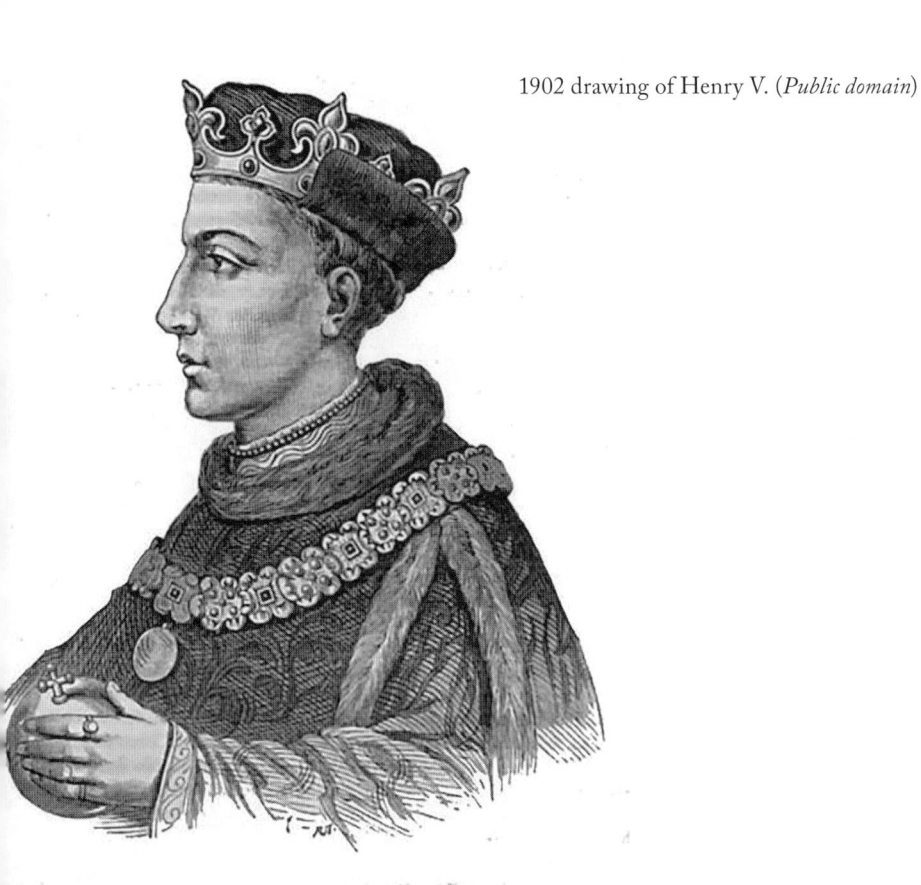

9th century drawing of the Battle of Bosworth. (*Public domain*)

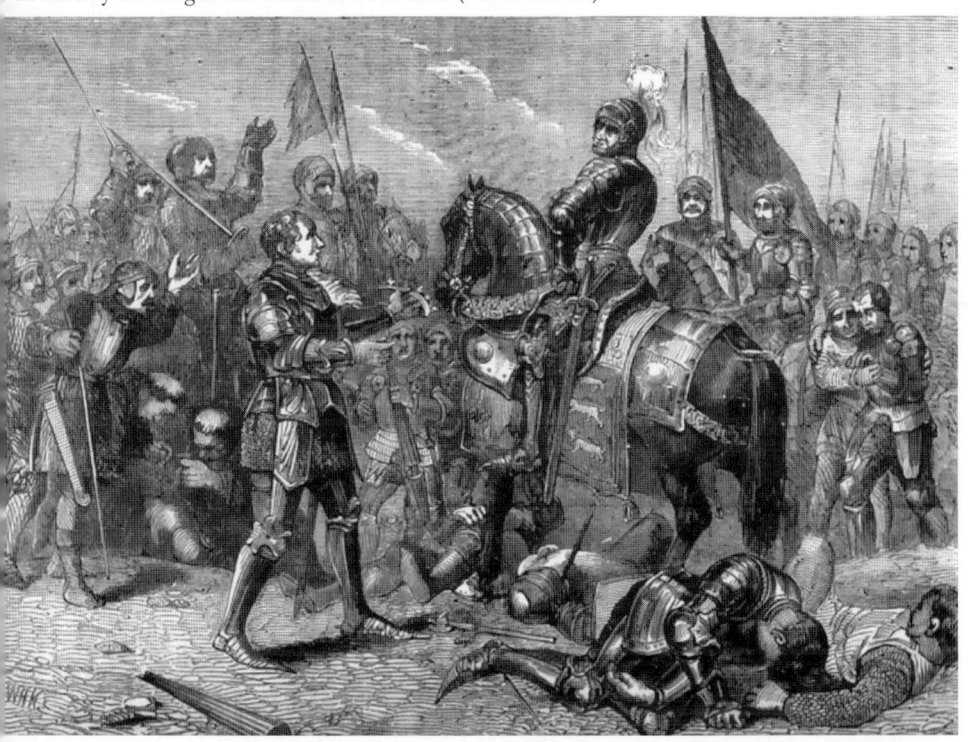

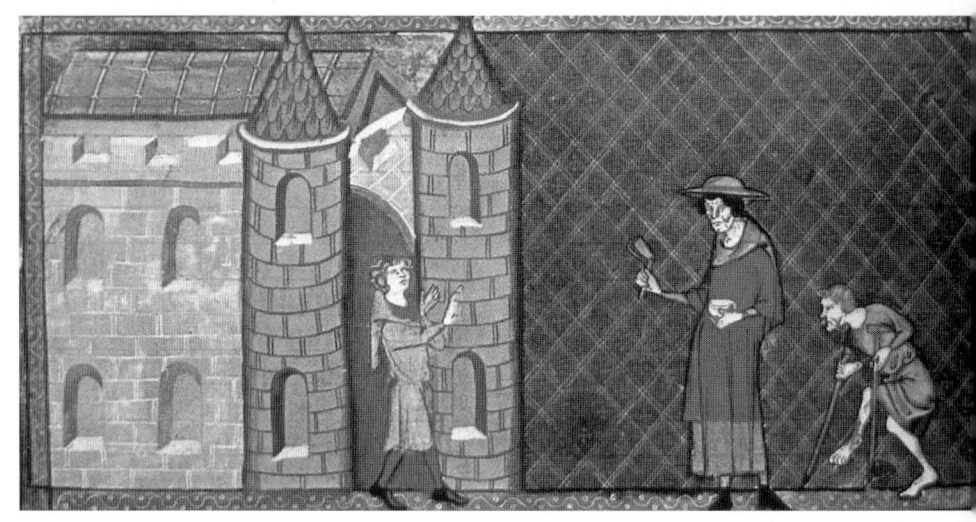

14th century drawing of the Leprosorium. (*Public domain*)

15th century drawing of patients at Hotel-Dieu in Paris. (*Public domain*)

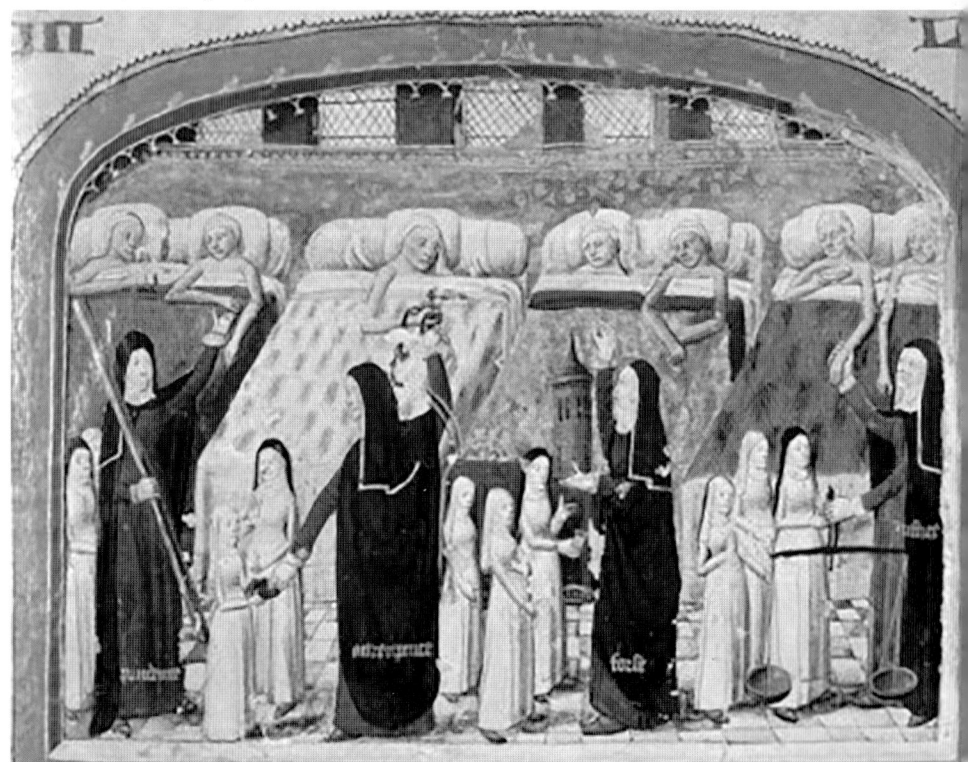

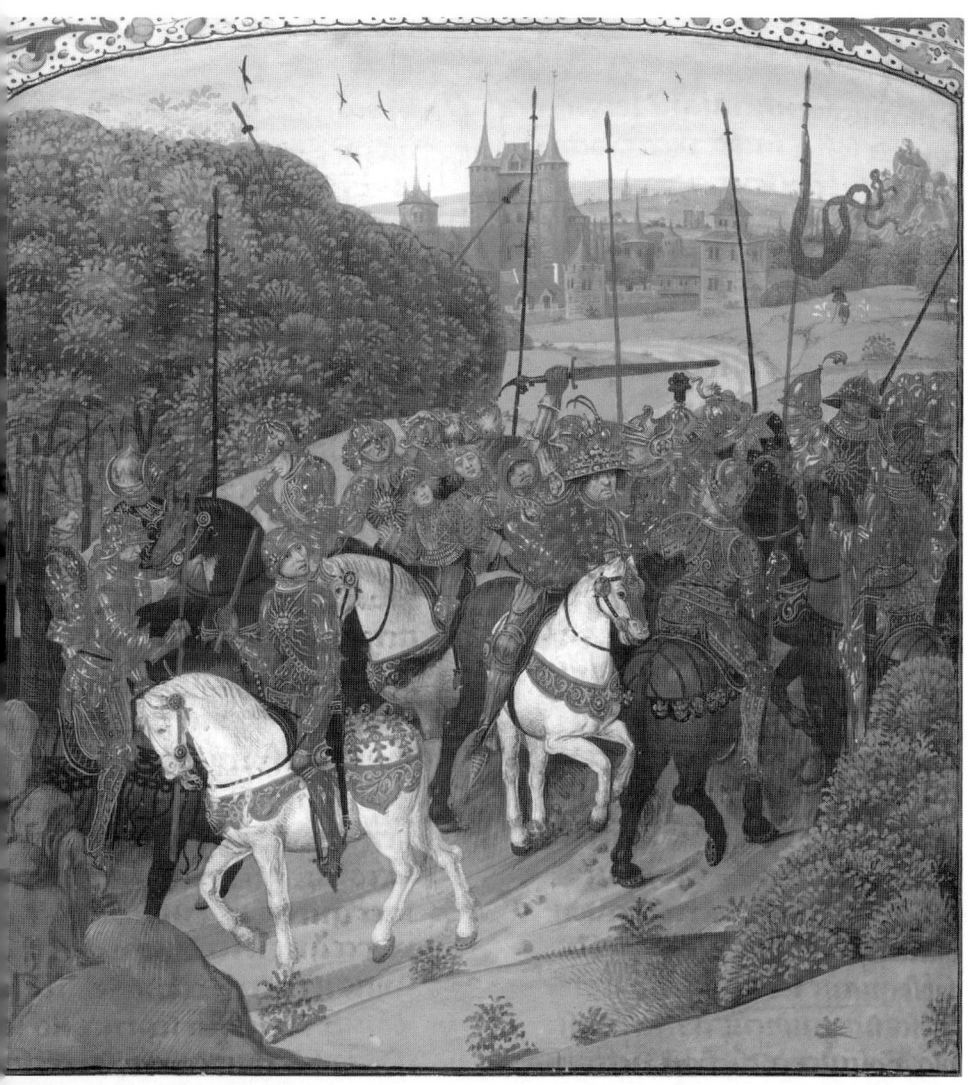

5th century painting depicting the madness of Charles V. (*Public domain*)

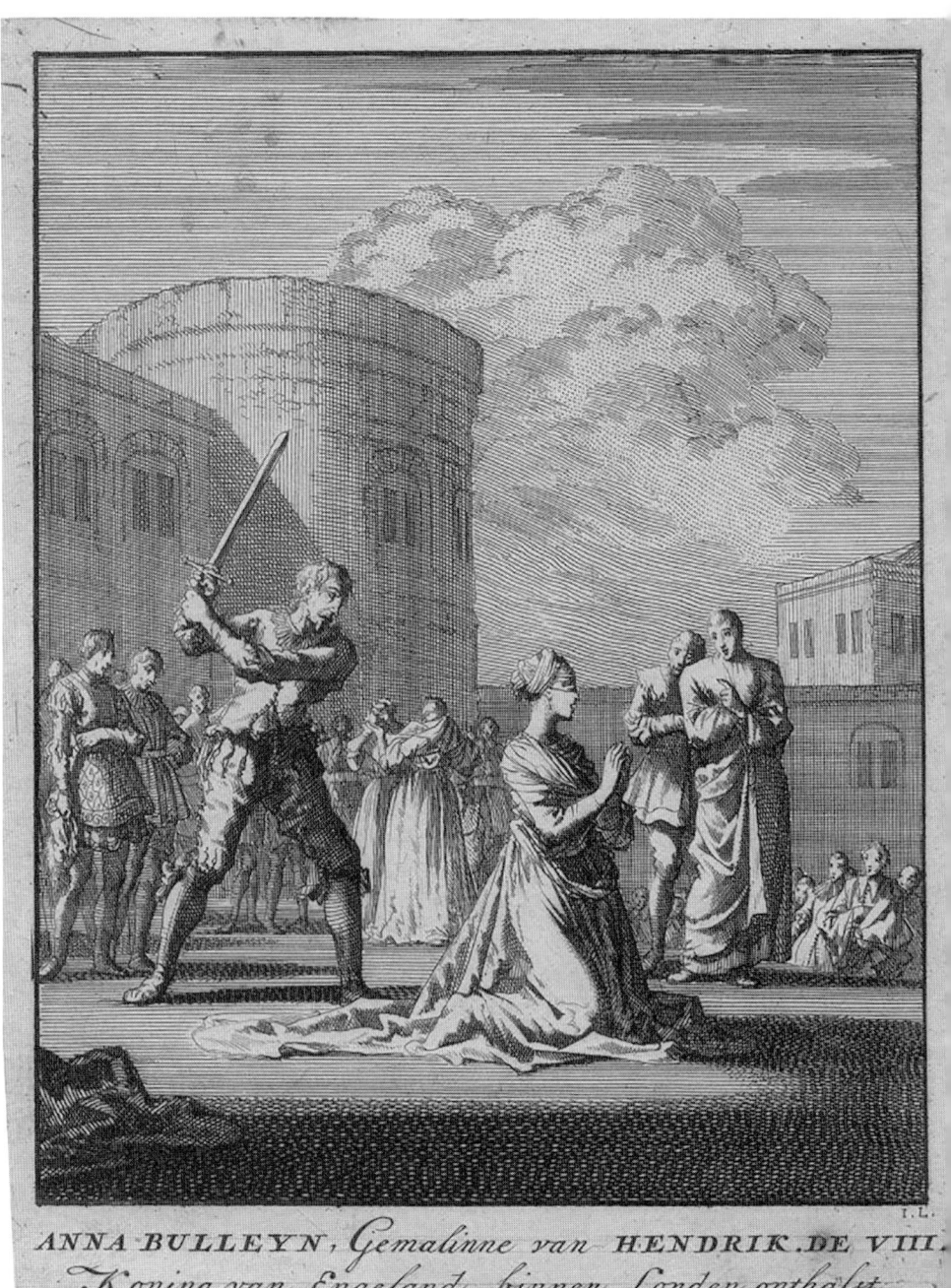

Anne Boleyn's execution. (*Public domain*)

in Ancient Egypt, was a tool that was used in assisting the midwife in a difficult delivery. The stool, shaped like a chair, enabled a labouring woman to sit upright with the help of her ladies. Her rear end would have been aligned with the opening at the bottom of the chair. This would have helped her adjust her pelvis enough so that the baby may have had an easier time making its way into the world. The stool was often padded for the mother's comfort, and it enabled the midwife to reach underneath to assist in delivering the child. Thanks to sterile surgical tools today, if a woman were to tear during childbirth or need an episiotomy, she would be given anaesthetic and antibiotics to prevent infection. During the Middle Ages, physicians were still unsure of what exactly had happened if the peritoneum broke. They suspected that part of the woman's womb was falling out.

The Sloane Manuscripts advised midwives to:

> Take good white wine, make it hot, add butter that is fresh. With the wine, moisten the womb until it gets supple and soft. Gently put it back where it should be. Then sew up the peritoneum in three or four places with double silken thread.

The midwife was then instructed to:

> Push linen cloth into the vulva and cover it with hot tar. Sit the patient upright in bed, so her feet are higher than her head, and let her remain there for nine days.

It is indeed hard for anyone reading this today to grasp the concept of why this advice was offered. Assuming that the baby had been delivered in this case, this procedure would again introduce a plethora of bacteria into the new mother's vagina. It also would have most likely left her with burns from the hot tar that was placed there afterwards. In the actual case of a prolapsed uterus, which appears to have been referred to as Precipitation of the Uterus, it was thought that when the uterus falls from its natural place to another place, this was because of "evil humours that are in the uterus" and:

> it falls out because of the illness that a woman has in bearing a child. If the uterus falls out underneath at the privy member after childbirth, let the midwife put it in again with her hands.

It was then advised to render such treatment as:

> Take the powder of gall, nutmeg, spikenard, and cloves and mix them together in a small linen bag and insert into the privy member to keep the uterus from falling out. Let it remain there for nine days. Let the patient eat and drink things that will not require her to go often to the privy or to urinate.

The Sloane Manuscript, when pertaining to the placenta, referred to it as *the secundine*. The teachings promised that if it was left behind after birth, it was because of a "great sickness of the mother's womb". It went onto explain this barbaric procedure as a way of requiring a midwife to deliver the afterbirth.

> The midwife should anoint her hands and with her nails, pull out the secundine if she can, and if she can't, bore holes in a stool and let the woman sit on it and make underneath a fumigation from goat's horns and claws of their feet so that the smoke strikes right up her privy member.

Assuredly this probably led to uterine infections. The Sloane Manuscript offered little to control any post-partum bleeding. It was advised, "do not give any comforting medicines, or baths, or medicated compresses". Instead, one was instructed to "have her bled under the ankle of one foot and another day under the other ankle".

Without the use of foetal scopes or ultrasound, it was impossible to be sure if a baby was stillborn. Guy de Chauliac offered that "contraction of the nipples, lack of movement in the womb, coldness, foulness of breath, sunken eyes and a lack of feeling in the lips and the face" in the mother may constitute a stillbirth. If the mother was unable to deliver her stillborn child, a midwife could "use a speculum to open the womb and draw the foetus out with hooks either in pieces or whole".

In the event that the mother had passed, but it was believed that the baby still thrived, de Chauliac instructed the midwife to "open the woman with a razor on the left side and put in the fingers and draw out the child".

There have been arguments among historians as to when the earliest caesarean sections were performed. Some will claim as early as in the year 3000 BCE in Egypt. But there is clear documentation that caesarean section births date back to Ancient Roman times. The name caesarean was initially believed to have been derived from the surgical delivery of Julius Caesar, but the theory that he was delivered via caesarean proves false. No woman would have survived such an ordeal, and the mother of Julius Caesar lived until sixty-five or sixty-six years of age. An early ancestor of Caesar may have been born caesarean. An early Roman law had been passed in 700 BCE, called *Lex Caesarea*, that stated a baby must be removed from a mother before she was buried, in the event she had died during childbirth. This was done because there was always a small chance that the baby may survive. This was the case with the later Church as well. In cases where the baby lived, but the mother did not, the Church wanted the baby removed and baptised immediately. Because a priest usually did this and a man was not allowed in the birthing room, in the fourteenth century, the Church authorised midwives to baptise babies in an event such as a caesarean section or an emergency. The first documented case in which a mother survived a caesarean section was believed to have taken place in 1337 in the city of Prague. Beatrice of Bourbon (1320–1383) was a French noblewoman who married King John of Bohemia (1296–1346) when she was only fourteen years old. In February 1337, Beatrice went into labour with her first child. Archival documents suggest that it was a difficult labour, and she likely fainted from exhaustion.

Believing that she had died, it was then that surgeons proceeded to open her belly to save the child. Of course, her doctors did not know about antiseptics, and any anaesthesia offered would have been insufficient. Any techniques used to stop bleeding or to clean the wound would have been archaic. A caesarean section meant almost certain death for the mother, either from the agony of surgery without anaesthesia or later from sepsis. In Beatrice's case, the pain from the operation likely caused her to awaken. Her doctors had probably cut her open in an attempt to baptize the baby and give it a chance at life. Medical knowledge today suggests that it may have been shock that kept her from bleeding to death. She certainly would have had the best royal doctors of the time as Prague was a modern centre of learning in Europe. A Flemish chronicle that was probably written by a diplomat at court said, "the duke was taken from his mother's body and the wound healed".

There isn't much more detailed evidence on the birth, but Beatrice recovered and lived out the rest of her life. Her son, Wenceslaus I, Duke of Luxembourg (1337–1383), lived to age forty-six.

If both a woman and her baby were lucky enough to survive the actual birth itself, it certainly didn't mean that either of them was out of the woods. Aside from eclampsia and haemorrhaging, women were at a very high risk for what was known as childbed fever. What we refer to today as puerperal fever, childbed fever, was a uterine infection that found its way into the bloodstream and eventually caused sepsis. This was a devastating condition, and it was genuine and terrifying. It usually started three to four days after the birth of the child and got continuously worse. Abdominal pain, fever, cold fits, sweating, thirst, and abdominal distention would plague the new mother as the days went on. Her resting pulse could get as high as 140 beats per minute. She became listless, with laboured breathing, nausea and vomiting, and sometimes delirium. Midwives and physicians knew the signs of childbed fever, and they also knew that there was a very good chance the mother wouldn't survive as it had a 70–80% morbidity rate.

Another person that knew the horrors of childbed fever was Henry VIII, as his own mother had died from it giving birth to his sister. And when his third wife, Jane Seymour (1508–1537), began to show the same signs days after the birth of their son, the king knew what to expect. Jane was a healthy, young queen at age 28 and had had a relatively trouble-free pregnancy. But when she went into labour, it would prove to be an extremely difficult delivery. Things didn't progress as the midwives had hoped, and Jane was in dire straits. The situation had become so bad that the king was asked if he wanted to save his wife or his child. It was possible that the baby wasn't in the correct birthing position, for Jane laboured for two days and three nights until at 2 am on 12 October 1537, she gave birth to a healthy baby boy. Queen Jane was utterly exhausted but appeared to be in good spirits. However, a few days later, she began to show signs of illness. Modern knowledge tells us that part of the placenta was left probably behind, and in her expended state of mind, Jane's body was more prone to infection. The dirty hands of midwives and soiled linens may have added to the problem. Jane continued to go downhill, and on 23 October, the king came to her bedside. Early in the morning on 24 October, after twelve days of immeasurable suffering, Queen Jane Seymour died of childbed fever.

It was around the fifteenth century that the Church began to mandate requirements around midwifery. Regulation of the trade became an ecclesiastical concern, and things began to change even more so after the Reformation. In 1535, Thomas Cromwell, chief minister to King Henry VIII, demanded that all relics and amulets be confiscated. The new Church of England was against superstition, and this included not only holy relics but pilgrimages as well. Prayer rolls were also taken, and it was instructed that labouring women pray directly to God himself. And although men were still not allowed in the room with the birthing mother unless there was an emergency, in the case of noble births, physicians would be close at hand. Queen Jane Seymour's doctors waited outside her door while she laboured and were there when things became dire.

The first year of a newborn's life during the Middle Ages was crucial. The odds were already stacked against them as there was a 50% chance they may not even survive the birth itself. Demography shows a very dark side of the lives of children. Less than 50% would live past the age of one, and roughly a quarter would live to age ten. Babies were breastfed well into their second year, usually by their mothers, unless they were of noble birth. But if a mother was sick herself and unable to nurse, the results could be devastating. Infants in medieval times, whether they came from a wealthy or poor family, spent the majority of their time being swaddled. While we still practise this today, it can be considered that swaddling an infant would help their arms and legs grow straight. Babies were wrapped up tight in linen cloth with their limbs tucked tightly to their sides. It most likely also provided somewhat of a safe haven for babies once they started moving around on their own. An infant that was swaddled in their cradle was at least protected from self-injury.

Medieval children of all ages were particularly vulnerable to an array of diseases, whether they were from infectious viruses or the high rate of bacteria due to unsanitary conditions. This applied especially to the children of people in the lower end of feudal society. Tuberculosis, dysentery, and sweating sickness could take the life of a child almost overnight. The nutrition of a child depended on their family's rank. Children of less wealthy families would most likely suffer from malnutrition. Not only did more impoverished families struggle to afford healthy foods, but it was actually believed that the stomachs of the poor could not handle foods rich in nutrients.

Children of serfs and families of peasants were looked upon as help around the home from an early age. Boys as young as the age of nine were expected to help in the fields doing hours of back-breaking work such as turning soil or helping to pull heavy farm machinery. Girls would often have to look after smaller siblings and would spend their days in the kitchen or tending to housework and sewing. Sadly, the work that children were made to do was probably responsible for their death in many cases. Accidents involving farming or hard labour often took the lives of boys or caused significant injury or dismemberment. Accidents with girls could arise around the fireplace or wells and most certainly in the kitchen.

If a child was born into a noble family, or more importantly, was the heir to the throne, there was much consideration put into keeping the child safe. Because of sickness or disease or power struggles in the court, a future king could often see his grave before he was old enough to wear the crown. Medieval marriages were not based on love; they were political unions that were designed to strengthen a country's alliance. Keeping the future heir to the throne safe was a critical job for those involved.

Once born, a noble child was taken under the care of a wet nurse for sustenance. Nursing a child, especially towards the later Middle Ages, was considered an inconvenience for a queen. As it was her job to produce healthy sons, it was the responsibility of the wet nurse to nourish them. Because breastfeeding usually provided natural birth control for at least six months, the Church was against it as well. The queen was expected to resume her political duties as soon as possible, and nursing a child was simply seen as an interruption. There are some tales, that although they remain sceptical, are intriguing. It is rumoured that at the birth of Princess Elizabeth in 1533, Anne Boleyn expressed a strong desire to nurse her own child but that the king forbade it.

A wet nurse for royal children was usually an appointed female who was well known throughout the household. The nurse had to have been someone with a healthy and wholesome diet, as it was thought that she passed on her own characteristics to the child she was nursing. She also had to be of youthful appearance and pleasant on the eyes, with clear skin and no imperfections. However, many parish records show that children who were not nursed by their own mothers tended to become ill or die. The reasoning behind this may have been that a wet nurse had to divide her attention, as well as her milk, to other children. Because the infant mortality rate was already high, this may have added to it.

But this didn't mean that wet nurses didn't care for other women's babies with less affection. Often wet nurses would remain members of the royal household where they became governess to the child and would stay with them throughout their childhood. While it may seem a bit cold-hearted to folks today to think of an infant being raised by someone other than its mother, it was done to keep the royal child free from infection and as healthy as possible. One such notable governess who had to undertake huge responsibility was Margaret Bryan (1468–1551). Lady Bryan was governess to all three of Henry VIII's children. She had been a lady in waiting to Katherine of Aragon, and upon the birth of Mary Tudor in 1516, she was appointed as her governess. She was also appointed governess to the king's daughter, Elizabeth, in 1533. While it was essential to watch over the lives of the two princesses, it was the prince who demanded the most attention. In 1537, she was appointed sole governess of Prince Edward (1537–1553), the king's long-awaited son. Henry demanded stringent codes of cleanliness for his son's household. Edward spent most of his early years at Hampton Court where the air was considered cleaner. The king lavished extreme care over the prince's apartments and ordered that they be cleaned daily.

Royal children were explicitly raised to carry out their family's heritage. Girls, primarily, were used as political pawns, and often a royal bride would be sent away for marriage in her teen years. Daughters of royals were traded to the highest bidder in the hopes that they too would carry on the family's legacy. The placement of young girls from noble families was to obtain the same objective. Like those women before them, their duty would have been to produce strong male heirs who could father more strong, healthy children.

Women in the Middle Ages should be looked upon heroically, for they performed the dangerous job of childbirth without thinking twice. And so, very often, they gave up their lives for the generation that followed in their footsteps.

Chapter Six

The Role of the Caretaker

In the spring of 1454, King Henry VI of England remained in the same general stupor he had been in since the previous August. In what seemed like a catatonic state, the king continued to alarm his council with his behaviour. He had become mute, almost unable to move, and completely void of his former self. The council assigned three doctors and two surgeons to his bedside to somehow treat and cure the king of his mysterious illness. In desperation, these five men would work together, bringing the best of their medical knowledge to the table. Ancient remedies that had stood the test of time, such as powders and syrups, would be tried along with enemas and ointments. The King would have been bled, his diet altered, all to save his life. But this wide range of treatment came from the different aspects of care that were believed to work. The king was fortunate to have physicians, surgeons, and apothecaries at his disposal. And like the barber-surgeon, each healer treated the body differently and had their own gifts to share.

Because of the sustained influence of Hippocrates and Galen, the Theory of Humourism would hold true to be the dominant theory in healing no matter if one was an astounding physician or a barber-surgeon still in training. Balance of the humours was the key to maintaining a healthy body and mind, and practitioners made it their mission to restore that balance when it fell by the wayside. Whether it involved diet, potions, or more aggressive approaches, the ultimate goal was the same, no matter the method.

The medieval physician was looked upon to assume responsibility for the inside of the body, including mental illness, such as in Henry VI's case. However, the surgeon played a different role in caring for the outside of the body. The surgeon might heal wounds or set broken bones, while the physician may turn to an apothecary to prepare an elixir of herbs to cure their patient. A barber-surgeon, while without a formal education, could perform simple surgeries or the removal of teeth. Looking back on these procedures today would most likely make one shudder, but I believe, for the most part, the intentions to heal were honest.

The medieval physician played a role unlike that of the surgeon, in where they rarely had to operate. The physician was responsible for curing the disease and for understanding what was going on inside of the body. Because of this, it was assumed that educated doctors should be learned at not only the inner workings of the body but those things that went on around it as well.

Educated doctors were encouraged to learn culture and art as well. They were expected to understand man's place in the world and the universe and to follow the humoral theory diet fully. Greek physicians believed that to do this, they needed to extend their knowledge past the human body. Greek physicians were not only that; they were philosophers. And to be highly respected, any medieval doctor must be one as well. Working almost exclusively in the service of the wealthy, physicians studied in Latin and were considered highly educated.

Most European universities caught on to this thought process and believed that students needed to have an additional two to three years of educational background in things other than medicine before they could graduate. Graduates, especially of Oxford and Cambridge, also had to be successful in the art of persuasive speaking and argument. These students were required to attend lectures on several different subjects, in addition to the teachings of Galen and Hippocrates.

As the Catholic Church began to gain dominance over the education system in the fourteenth and fifteenth centuries, theology seemed to be the only field of study they would support. More and more universities made a push for studying theology, and focusing on anything else was much frowned upon by the Church. Between the years 1300 and 1499, only fifty-nine students graduated with a medical degree. In the fifteenth century, Oxford university handed out 500 theology degrees and only forty degrees in medicine.

John Gaddesden (1280–1361) was an English physician who began his studies at Merton College, Oxford, in 1299. Starting in 1305, he wrote a medical treatise titled *Rose Anglica*, or *Practical Medicine from Head to Foot*. The book goes over accounts of fever and disease, diagnosis through urine, and several remedies and prescriptions. The *Rose Anglica* became one of the first English textbooks of medicine. It was through this book that Henry VI was given a course of therapy for his forgetfulness and confusion. John of Gaddesden recommended the following to restore clarity and to expel evil humours:

> It is necessary for lethargic that people talk loudly in their presence. Tie their extremities lightly and rub their palms and soles hard, and let their feet be put in saltwater up to the middle of their shins, and pull their hair and nose, and squeeze the toes and fingers tightly, and cause pigs to squeal in their ears; give them a sharp clyster at the beginning, and open the vein of the head, or nose, or forehead, and draw blood from the nose with the bristles of a boar. Put a feather, or a straw, in his nose to compel him to sneeze, and do not ever desist from hindering him from sleeping; and let human hair or other evil-smelling thing be burnt under his nose. Apply, moreover, the cupping horn between the shoulder, and let a feather be put down his throat to cause vomiting, and shave the back of the head, and rub oil of roses and vinegar and wild celery juice thereon.

Gaddesden chose the name *Rose Angelica* because he likened it to the five sepals of a rose. Sepals are the support system for the petals of a flower, and because the rose outshined all other flowers, he believed his book outshined all other text on the practice of medicine. His book is rich with ideas from Galen, Avicenna, and Averroes, as well as other pioneering minds of medicine. He also filled the pages of *Rosa Angelica* with remarks on cooking and remedies. It was printed several times, in Pavia in 1492, in Venice in 1502, and again in Augsburg in 1595. Gaddesden was appointed to the stall of Wildland in St. Paul's Cathedral in the year 1342, twenty years before his death.

Uroscopy, a method of determining one's ailment through their urine, became extremely common during the Middle Ages. The first records of uroscopy date back to Ancient Greek and Indian times. Hippocrates believed that urine was a result of the four humours, and this led Galen to put his own spin on the belief. He refined that one's urine was a filtered result of one's blood only and not bile or phlegm. Studying urine eventually reached the Byzantine empire and became the main focus of diagnosing an ailment.

Further inspiration was found by other cultures, predominantly Arab and Jewish scholars. Still, despite these findings, uroscopy was mostly maintained by the teachings of Hippocrates and Galen when it reached the west. Perhaps because it was socially unacceptable to examine a patient, for the most part, the observation of their urine would help the doctor to diagnose illness. Medieval doctors believed that looking at urine could examine the health of the liver, where they thought blood was made. They would interpret the colour of the patient's urine by comparing it to the Urine Wheel, which showed a rainbow of colours that urine could be. The colours on the wheel went from bright white to various shades of yellow to black. Doctors and barber-surgeons would examine urine in a glass flask, known as a *matula* that had a rounded bottom. Holding it up to the light, physicians studied the appearance, smell, and even the taste of the urine. They believed these aspects were all equally important as they corresponded to the colours on the urine wheel. The wheel was much like a diagram that linked the colour of the patient's urine to particular diseases. Temperature was also critical when making a diagnosis. The urine had to stay warm to be adequately evaluated because when the temperature decreased, impurities would be more challenging to read due to the settling of bubbles. Letting urine cool also caused it to be thicker, which would lead to a false diagnosis. So, urine was typically analysed right away, in proper lighting. Lighting could not be too bright or too dark as this would not allow the physician to see the urine correctly.

The iconic image of the creepy plague doctor, dressed in his long black gown, with the beak-like mask stuffed with herbs, comes to mind when one thinks of the physicians who treated those with the plague. But these cane wielding medical men didn't wear these creepy costumes until the seventeenth century. Plague doctors wore these masks to protect them from being infected as they believed the disease was airborne. To battle this miasma or bad air, the long beak of the mask was stuffed with sweet-smelling herbs and dried flowers, but there is no evidence that the costume and mask were worn during the fourteenth-century outbreak. The outfit was designed in 1619 by a French doctor named Charles de Lorme (1548–1678) as a form of head-to-toe protection. Plague doctors were explicitly hired by town officials in towns where the plague had taken hold. They were to treat everyone, both rich and poor, but these "doctors" were usually not experienced physicians or surgeons at all. They were typically substandard, unsuccessful doctors or young physicians who were just getting their feet wet and needed to establish themselves. Many community plague doctors were untrained, lacking any medical training at all, and often gave an educated guess while giving their diagnosis and treatment. Whether experienced physicians were not available or simply were too afraid to treat patients is unknown. It's possible that since university-trained physicians generally limited their practice to those on the upper rung of society, they simply were not available. But whatever the reason, there was a considerable rise in the number of unlicensed and untrained practitioners during the plague.

The plague of 1348 was a time of desperation. Doctors whose sole purpose was to treat this killer often knew little more than their patients. Poultices of onion and butter, arsenic, and floral components were just no match. History tells us of some rather ridiculous methods used by doctors for treating the plague. Bloodletting was used in the hopes that being bled would expel bad humours. Incisions were often made near the bubo itself, which of course caused nothing more than further infection. Cutting the bubo open and draining it of the foul-smelling pus was a technique used by Guy de Chauliac. When the black death reached Avignon, physicians fled the city. But de Chauliac stayed, treating patients and documenting their treatment as he went along. He became infected himself but somehow managed to survive, unlike Italian doctor Gentile da Foligno, who passed in June 1348 after also treating plague victims. Patients were also given herbal treatment that would cause increased sweating as it was believed that raising the temperature of the body would help the patient to sweat out the disease. Theriac, as described later in the chapter, was used to rid the body of the plague. The syrup from refined sugar was fed to the patients in the hopes that it would help to rid the body of the disease. It's certainly possible that mould spores with disease-fighting properties may have developed over the ten years that theriac had to be stored. Yet it is doubtful that it saved many lives. Doctors believed that bathing in urine offered relief of plague symptoms, and some even encouraged their patients to drink it. Patients of more well-to-do families were given a paste made from water and crushed emeralds to swallow. It was considered that the crushed stones would restore the humours to balance. Pastes were also made from human faeces and mixed with flour and tree resin. Buboes were then cut open and the paste was smeared inside and covered with a bandage. Because doctors believed that dinner parties would reduce stress and cause one to be merry, they actually encouraged the idea of gathering together. But we now know that this was probably the worst thing they could have done.

Doctors who treated the plague were very valuable and often given exclusive rights. They were freely allowed to conduct autopsies on deceased patients, in search of a cure. This undoubtedly gave them much credit, as autopsies were otherwise forbidden during the fourteenth century. It seemed that physicians responded to the Black Death in one of two ways. Many wrote several treatises of the plague, lecturing on the ways it could be prevented or to offer cures to alleviate its effects, or writing on ways to tackle the issue head-on instead of speculating about its origins. At the request of King Philip VI (1293–1530) of France, the faculty at the University of Paris devised a treatise on the possible reasons behind the plague. It also offered advice on how to avoid contracting it. This writing suggested that the wrath of God, along with the conjunction of the planets, had caused the plague. The text offered suggestions on how to avoid getting ill by "Choosing air as clean and pure as possible; dry, with no mixtures of corrupting vapours".

It was instructed that:

Inhabitants should leave any place where and in which the air is mixed with corrupting vapours, if possible. If not, they should choose a dwelling place away from the wind channels that carry thee corrupt vapours, as in humid houses, where the air is stagnant.

When it came to exercise, the treatise says, "As long as the air is calm, those who are in the habit of exercising should do a little less than normal so that they do not intensify the need to breathe". It also cautioned to:

avoid taking a hot bath because it relaxes and moistens the body. A hot bath should be rare and rarer still for those whose body is replete. Only those who are strongly habituated to it and those with a fat and compact build can do it to moisten themselves in trying to expel the sickness

Abu Ja'far Ahmad Ibn Khatima, a Muslim doctor living in Almeria, Spain, speaks of the Black Death from his first-hand experience with the epidemic. Khatima's work is one of the most detailed accounts in history, and it's interesting to look at his methods of treatment in contrast to the Christian ones. Aside from discussing practical remedies, Khatima also offered concrete treatments for the plague. He believed that therapy for a plague victim should start with being bled after giving the patient a mixture of vinegar and syrup. He felt that the patient should be bled from whatever area they felt the most pain and the bleeding was to continue until the patient felt weak. He watched closely for the patient's fever to fall and then gave a mixture of apple and lemon syrups with rose water and vinegar. This was followed by a peppermint broth and then by sour pomegranate. There were hopes that the patient would recover, along with having to be bled from time to time to be sure all the toxins were removed from the body. But if the sickness continued for more than two days or was followed by the spitting up of blood or vomit, there was little hope for the patient at this point. If the patient was still alive after the seventh day, Khatima gave instructions to open any buboes that had filled with pus. He said it was essential to wait for the buboes to be ripe for opening. It would be terrible for a patient to suffer a relapse after lancing. Remedies were then prescribed to ease the irritation caused by draining the buboes.

Like Khatima, Gentile would also begin his treatments with bleeding a patient to the point of weakness. He then recommended placing a cup over any buboes and opening them with a knife on the second day of the illness. Gentile suggested that the buboes be cauterised and covered with a plaster to draw out the poison. And like Khatima, he also offered remedies to be given to the patient to help him regain his strength. But it was Gentile who really had the best solution of all, and it was simply to leave the infected areas alone. Gentile had grown frustrated with the lengthy discussions that were being had by physicians as he felt that what really mattered was the treatment. He believed that it did not matter what caused the sickness, only what would be done about it. He wrote in regard to this opinion:

> As for those wishing to extinguish a fire burning a house, it is enough to know that it is a fire, that it may not destroy us, whether it be produced by fire or by motion; and for those wishing to resist the poisonous bite of a dry asp, it is enough to know that the asp was biting, whether it was generated by coition or from putrefaction.

For it had become evident that merely theorizing over the plague was not sufficient in dealing with it. The works of Hippocrates, Galen, and Avicenna simply did not provide medieval practitioners with enough information on how to combat something as substantial as the plague. In no way had their works prepared doctors for the task that lay before them in 1348.

In the beginning stages of syphilis, many treatments were not only ineffective but downright dangerous. Medical professionals that treated syphilis with bloodletting, laxatives, and sweat baths would help to rid the body of the disease-causing substance. Physicians believed that the induction of sweating and salivating would help to eliminate the poisons as well. Guaiacum, a flowering plant, was used in the treatment of syphilis in the early sixteenth century. Italian physician Girolamo Fracastoro (1476–1553) describes the use of guaiacum in his 1530 poem, *Syphilis, Sive Morbus Gallicus*:

> in external use for dressing ulcers, abscesses and pustules. For internal use drink the first potions by the beaker twice a day; in the morning at sunrise and by the light of the evening star. The treatment lasts until the moon completes its orbit and after the space of a month conjoins again with the sun. The patient must remain in a room protected from wind and cold so that frost and smoke do not diminish the effect of the remedy.

Using guaiacum didn't harness the unpleasant side effects of its counterpart in treatment, but it wasn't terribly effective either. Swiss doctor Paracelsus (1493–1541) was one of the first supporters of using mercury as a treatment for syphilis as it had positive effects on leper patients in the Arabic world. Doctors had reason to believe that the two diseases were related. Paracelsus also described the use of guaiacum as useless and expensive. Although he favoured the use of mercury for medicinal treatments, it wasn't until after a time that he understood the toxicity of the product. Mercury treatment could be administered as a drink. After realising this wasn't the safest method, Paracelsus resorted to using it as an ointment to be rubbed on the skin. A patient that was about to undergo this treatment was taken to a warm room and rubbed with an ointment containing mercury several times a day. This was done next to a fire, and the patient was then to stay close to the fire to sweat profusely. This treatment could carry on for months and continuously be repeated if little improvement was seen. He also advocated for the inhalation of mercury while bathing the body in the hot, steamy water.

However, using mercury therapy invited a whole host of horrific side effects. Kidney failure, mouth ulcers, and loss of one's teeth, as well as full-blown mercury poisoning, would often kill the patient before the disease had a chance to. Because treatment carried on for years sometimes, it gave rise to the saying "A night with Venus, and a lifetime with mercury". Because the effects of syphilis were so disfiguring, I feel it is only fair to give an honourable mention to Italian facial surgeon Gaspare Tagliacozzi (1545–1599). Although his work is much past the time of the Middle Ages, his pioneering work was one of the earliest attempts at reconstructing the nose defects caused by syphilis. Tagliacozzi understood that blood supply was crucial to being able to harvest nearby tissue for its use. His technique took tissue from the upper arm without removing its vital blood supply. This meant that the patient remained with their arm strapped to their face for quite some time in the hopes that new blood vessels would grow at the site of the damage. Ultimately, if it went according to plan, then the new flap could be separated from the arm during a second procedure.

As in the case of several monarch physicians, the role of university-trained doctors often took on more than just that; they became dieticians, spiritual counsellors, and confidants, in addition to being an actual physician. But one thing physicians weren't, were surgeons. University of Paris graduates in 1350, and going forward, swore an oath that they would never attempt any kind of manual surgery. The fear of accidentally killing a patient was just too great. Many physicians felt great restraint and grew too fearful of practising anything beyond preventative medicine. A doctor's career could be at stake if he were to be sued for wrongful death, and many doctors embraced the English theory, that scholastic training could be more beneficial.

The first duty of any doctor in royal or ecclesiastical service was to the patron himself. Although the pay was usually higher, sometimes the requests were a bit out of line, and physicians were expected to be at the beck and call of their masters. Some doctors preferred to work on more of a per diem basis rather than give their undivided attention to one person or family. While payments from royalty were in the form of not only cash but jewels, plates, and expensive clothes, it didn't necessarily mean that a physician was ready to subject all his time to serving just one patient. But in the case that one was appointed to the monarchy, they often had little choice.

Such an example lay with the medical staff of King Edward IV (1442–1483), as they were passionate about keeping him safe from leprosy as well as keeping anyone away from him that may have had the dreaded disease. In 1486, as part of their plan to be sure they knew if anyone had an accurate diagnosis, three of the king's doctors, who were men of the "arts and physics", examined a suspected leprosy victim. The doctors were extremely thorough in their examination of her, and by the fifteenth century, these types of scrutinizing looks were becoming more of a regular thing. Senior members of the medical team who were learned men were asked to seek out victims of leprosy to keep the monarchy safe. And Edward's doctors, like all doctors of the crown, went above and beyond the call of duty to ensure the safety of their monarch.

The physical decline of King Henry VIII kept many court doctors in attendance and well paid. When Henry came to the throne in 1509, he was good-looking and athletic. Tall at six foot two, he had broad shoulders and muscular arms and legs. His piercing blue eyes and red hair made him the most handsome prince in all of Christendom. The king was a passionate sportsman and enjoyed sports including tennis, hunting, and jousting. But starting in his early thirties, he began to encounter a series of unfortunate medical events that would slowly bring him down. At a jousting tournament, the king forgot to put his visor down, and his opponent struck him in the head above his right eye. The blow began a progression of terrible headaches that would affect him for the rest of his life. Because of the tight hose worn during Tudor times, the king started to suffer from varicose ulcers. The king's muscular calves were the talk of his kingdom, and he always made an effort to show them off with his hose. After his jousting accident in 1536, the king began his steady decline into poor health. He was forty-four years old, and being thrown from his horse, in full armour with the horse falling on top of him, caused the wounds in his leg to worsen. Aside from the head injury caused by the fall, the pain from his ulcers, made his life quite miserable at times.

Thomas Vicary (1490–1561) was one of the king's court doctors. Because of his success in treating the king's leg wound, Vicary was advanced to the position of sergeant-surgeon to the Royal Household. The worsening of the king's leg left him unable to participate in the sports that he loved so much. He developed ulcers on both legs that became constantly infected and omitted a horrible smell. Vicary and his other court physicians tried to keep the wounds open to allow drainage of the humours and often lanced the ulcers with red hot pokers. The king's mood was foul since his head injury and the death of his third wife, Queen Jane. No doubt that a therapy like the one provided for his leg wounds would have worsened his ill-temper.

In the 1540 portrait, *Granting of the Charter to the Barber-Surgeons*, by artist Hans Holbein (1497–1543), Vicary stands next to the king along with his other prominent court physicians, John Chambre (1470–1549) and Sir William Butts (1486–1545). Dr Butts was the premier royal physician to the king as well as other members of his court. He was a trusted member of Henry's circle and one of the only men the king trusted. Dr Butts was paid well by the king, and his pay continued to increase. He was physician to Princess Mary at Ludlow Castle, and when the king's sweetheart Anne Boleyn fell ill with the sweating sickness, it was Dr Butts that he sent to care for her. Butts was also physician to young Prince Edward, the most important person in the king's life. When the prince fell ill with fever in 1541, Butts was sent to oversee his care. He was adamant that the prince followed a diet of hot broths and soups and stayed with him while he recovered over a matter of days. During his marriage to Anne of Cleves (1515–1557) in 1540, the king confided in Dr Butts about his concerns that he was impotent. But the doctor reassured him that the fault lay with the queen, who could not "excite and provoke any lust in him".

The constant fear of death and illness during the Middle Ages often placed patients at their doctor's mercy. Physicians became personal, trusted advisors, and close relationships grew between the two. But unfortunately, many physicians were nothing more than certified quacks, preying on people who were desperate to feel better. Folks who might present with disgusting skin diseases that they feared may have been leprosy found themselves going to a doctor less trustworthy. Often, these unfortunate people ended up spending more money on nothing but a bogus cure.

Physicians with integrity felt that each individual symptom of a disease should be treated as a disease of the humours in itself. But once doctors began to treat people, they may have started to realize that what they were taught in medical school was not always the best approach. Physicians began to realise that they learned better through experience, along with academic text containing a mixture of remedies applied with theoretical principles of medicine. As a first step towards a cure, a physician may suggest a medication that may soften the heat or the cold of the affected part of the body. By using a medicinal preparation that generated natural heat when applied, physicians were also hopeful that the body could be encouraged to defend itself against harmful humours. While plasters, ointments, and salves were commonly used for skin diseases, they were also applied in the event of severe internal disorders. These ointments could either encourage or prevent the loss of heat and moisture in the body, thus allowing it to recover its humoral balance.

When it came to cleansing the body with a more hands-on approach, one turned to the medieval surgeon. Whether it was ridding the body of unwanted humours through induced vomiting or defecation, in cases of severe or acute illness, some things were out of reach of preventative medicine. Physicians worked alongside surgeons to prescribe medications and remedies but left the act of performing manual operations to the surgeon.

John of Arderne (1307–1392), who attended the University of Montpellier in France, was an English surgeon, who was one of the first of his time to formulate functional cures. He is considered to be one of the fathers of surgery and is still remembered today for his pioneering in medicine. He felt strongly that a patient should feel no cutting during a procedure, and he experimented with opium and soporific as a way to induce sleep for his patients before an operation. John of Arderne devised several different concoctions of enemas that he felt were helpful in the treatment of constipation. A mixture of the mallow plant, water, green chamomile, salt, wheat bran, honey, herbs, and a mild soap was recommended to be squirted into the rectum via a greased pipe to ease discomfort. The tube was usually attached to a bag made of the bladder of an animal, primarily a pig. He also advised hot baths in scented water to ease constipation and stomach pain. He believed that the steaming water would also expel impurities such as fever or bladder stone. He was also known for developing several treatments for knights for painful cysts that would develop due to hard riding in the saddle. The affliction, *Fistula in*

Ano, caused a large, painful lump at the base of the spine and anus. What is known today as a pilonidal cyst, *Fistula in Ano* was an abscess that, once ruptured, could become a fistula. This was an extremely painful ailment, and to have it drained must have given the knights much relief. Arderne was successful in cutting the offending lump and bandaging it along with an ointment made from hemlock, opium, and henbane. John of Arderne was admitted as a member of the Guild of Surgeons in 1370 in London and referred to himself as Master Surgeon in his own works.

Perhaps the most popular surgical procedure of restoring balance to the humours was bloodletting. Bloodletting was believed to rid the body of excess humours. It was used not only as an acute treatment but also as a preventative for those who were feared to become ill. Bloodletting was regarded as a fundamental treatment during the later Middle Ages and became so popular that there was the problem of unqualified people performing the procedure. Considered to be one of medicine's oldest practices, bloodletting would involve the opening of a vein by a surgeon with a lancet or other sharp object. This would cause the blood to flow out into a waiting receptacle in hopes of a sign of relief from the patient. Greek physician Erasistratus believed that every illness came from an excess accumulation of blood. Galen expanded on this theory, and it found its way into India and the Arab world as well.

Bloodletting soon became the custom of religious houses and priories, as well as treatment for the sick. The Augustinian Priory of Barnwell in Cambridgeshire bled their brothers on average seven times a year. It's recorded that they were able to rest and eat a well-balanced meal after being bled. Perhaps this is why they reported feeling better after being bled, and not because of the actual bloodletting itself. Other priories bled their brothers as often as every six weeks and built special wings that were intended for just this very thing. Doctors felt that, along with a proper diet, bleeding priory members was necessary for the prevention of illness.

A fourteenth century drawing entitled *Vein Man* goes into great detail about where a vein should be opened. The picture is part of *The Guildbook of Barber-Surgeons of York* and diagrams nineteen points on the body for drawing blood. The drawing of a naked man illustrates what veins can be used and when. The text that accompanies the picture goes into specifics and brings the number of entry points on the body to thirty-three. The diagram makes clear the reasoning behind each operation, such as piercing the area between the finger and thumb to ease the pain of a headache or migraine. For diseases of the bladder, a vein in the ankle should be opened. For leprosy, two veins in the "neck hole". This diagram, as well as others that illustrated bloodletting, explained that blood was often bled from the arms and legs, usually below the elbow. Bleeding from this point not only cleared the liver and spleen but was also used as a preventative treatment.

The popularity of bloodletting didn't mean that all surgeons were necessarily on board with the procedure. By the eleventh and twelfth centuries, the leading works of Jewish and Arab medical authorities were becoming more available. Isaac Judaeus, believed to have lived between 832 and 932, was one of the most notable Jewish physicians residing in the Arab world at the time. He had his reservations about bloodletting and believed it was rather foolish to draw blood from someone if it wasn't necessary. Robert Burton (1577–1640), a scholar at Oxford University, thought that bloodletting was downright dangerous and only made humoral imbalance worse. He believed it caused blindness and depression and did nothing to help the patient.

English doctors understood that bloodletting could be fatal and people often bled to death at the hands of careless surgeons. In 1278, a trial was held for a patient named William le Paumer, who had collapsed and died as a result of a bloodletting procedure gone wrong. The doctor had accidentally severed an artery, and le Paumer bled to death. Unfortunately, the trial brought no justice, as no physicians were found at fault for his death.

Perhaps it is more reassuring to know that some surgeons in the Middle Ages understood that bleeding a pregnant or menstruating woman, children, or the elderly was too risky. But because they still truly believed that some form of phlebotomy was the ultimate line of defence, there were other ways to "bleed" a patient without actually cutting them. Surgeons understood that they could bleed a patient who was too weak by the use of leeches.

The European Medicinal Leech, *Hirudo medicinalis*, was nothing more than an aquatic bloodsucking worm. But it was quite a valuable tool in medicine throughout history because of its many medicinal uses. The first documented evidence of using leeches dates back before Galen, but he too was an advocate of bleeding patients with them. The saliva of a leech contains a substance that would anaesthetise the wound area and dilate blood vessels, increasing blood flow to the area. Leeches, who were usually gathered by a designated leech collector, were found in clear, running streams. They were typically starved for a day while being kept in clean water. Surgeons placed leeches on open wounds, ulcers, haemorrhoids, or boils to draw blood to the surface of the skin. Aside from being a less painful alternative to bloodletting by way of the knife, leeches also posed less of a risk of infection.

Another less invasive alternative to traditional phlebotomy or bloodletting was cupping. The act of cupping, believed to date back over 3000 years ago, involved placing heated glass or brass over skin that had been braised or scratched with a knife or sharp tool. By doing so and adding a suction-like action over the wound, it stimulated a gentle flow of blood towards the surface of the skin. Cupping was usually confined to the neck area to treat blemishes around the eyes, mouth, or face. It was used near the shoulders if one was believed to have a chest infection or near the lower back and buttocks if it was a liver ailment that plagued you. Cupping could alleviate arthritis by being practised on the upper arms or placed on the thighs in the event of bladder or reproductive organ troubles. Used on or near the stomach, cupping could help to ease an upset stomach. To relieve a blocked nose, simply treat the area about the head. While cupping is still in use today, it had been deemed pseudoscience or a celebrity fad. And it probably did nothing more than result in bruising, burns, and possible infections. Patients were often left with excessive fluid accumulation in the tissues and ruptured blood vessels, but given the alternative of bloodletting, it was still deemed safer during the Middle Ages.

The history of cauterisation has been documented in the Hippocratic Corpus and today remains an effective method of removing unwanted tissue. Surgeons during the Middle Ages understood that heating specific instruments to the right temperature could be useful in removing dead tissue and healing wounds. It was also effective in stopping excess bleeding. The humoral theory taught surgeons that cauterisation eliminated cold and moist humours that were responsible for headaches and seizures, as well as disorders of the throat and ears. Al-Zahrawi (936–1013), an Arab surgeon who was considered the most exceptional surgeon of the Middle Ages, believed that cauterisation had a use for everything. Al-Zahrawi's book, *Kitab-al-Tasrif*, a thirty-volume work on medical practice, was translated into Latin and used in European medicine over the next 500 years. Al-Zahrawi specialised in cauterisation and developed surgical devices that were used to inspect the urethra and how to remove foreign objects from the throat. Following a course of laxatives, Al-Zahrawi described a procedure for getting rid of excessive humidity and coldness from the brain:

> bid the patient open the bowels with an evacuant, which will also clear his head, for three or four nights, according to the strength, age, and habits of the patient. Then tell him to have his head shaved; then seat him cross-legged before you, with his hands on his breast. Then place the lower part of your palm upon the root of his nose between his eyes, and where your middle finger reaches, mark that place with ink. Then heat an olivary cautery. Then bring it down upon the marked placed with one downward stroke with gentle pressure, revolving the cautery; then quickly take your hand away while observing the place. If you see that some bone is exposed, the size of the head of a skewer or a grain of vetch, then take your hand away; otherwise, repeat with the same iron or, if that has gone cold, with another, till the amount of bone I have mentioned is exposed. Then take a little salt in water; soak some cotton in it, apply to the place, then leave for three days.

The shape of cauterising tools would indicate how to treat certain things and the instrument needed to be so hot that it gave off sparks. Al-Zahrawi prided himself on taking surgery and cauterisation seriously as he understood that things could go very wrong. He understood the ramifications of not doing so and knew that, at times, cauterisation could do more harm than good. This was certainly the case in a twelfth-century attempt in Iceland to cauterise a patient's stomach wound. The cauterising tool was said to have plunged into the patient's stomach. As it was recorded in the miracle book of the patron saint of Iceland, Porlakr Porhallsson, "a great bursting sound that occurred when the lesser membrane that was situated in the intestine burst apart...fat flowed from it, which they believed was from the intestine".

The practice of cataract surgery, also known as couching, began quite surprisingly in Ancient Greece and Ancient India. It was used well into the Middle Ages, in a procedure in which the surgeon would attempt to dislodge the cloudy lens by forcing a blunt object into the eye. The purpose was to break the cataract up and push it to the bottom of the eyeball. However, this procedure was far from beneficial; it was ineffective and extremely dangerous. Over 70% of people who had the operation performed on them went blind, making their situation that much worse.

When it came to illustrations of medieval surgery, the agony and discomfort that patients felt were much overlooked. Drawings depicted happy and serene patients, who paid no mind to the fact that they were being butchered without anaesthesia. Most herbal remedies that were used in Western medicine were not reliable, and some were even deadly. Doctors had absolutely no understanding of dosage. All they understood was that the drugs were "designed to reduce the body's natural heat through agents that had a coldness". Physician John of Arderne did recommend several preparations for pain relief, but understandably, many surgeons were weary of their risk. Cocktails made of opium or hemlock could be fatal, and oddly some of these were found in home remedy books as well as in actual medical books for surgeons. One recipe for such a cocktail, or dwale, was gall from a castrated sow or boar, lettuce, briony vine, opium, juice of hemlock, and wine. This concoction surely would have knocked a patient entirely out of it and caused them to defecate themselves as well and one tiny slip up in the dosage of this anaesthetic could kill you. Even with "anaesthesia" at a proper dosage, surgeons had to operate quickly. There was no understanding of how to slow the loss of blood which would promptly do damage to the organs. And once heavy bleeding began, it was difficult to stop. Surgeons attempted to use a styptic, which was an anti-haemorrhaging agent, usually made up of egg whites, gum, frankincense, aloe, and hair, to stop bleeding and encourage tissue to clot. But without the use of modern medicine, internal haemorrhaging would likely take your life, no matter how you chose to try and stop it. More often than not, it was a losing battle to save a patient once it was evident the end was near.

Medieval surgeons certainly understood that what they were doing was overall dangerous and at times wondered if it was worth the risk. Not only legally but knowing that they may have caused a death or mutilation most likely put tremendous strain on them both personally and professionally. Because of the Church's influence, being the cause of one's death would have caused surgeons to ponder how they might be viewed in both the eyes of the clergy and the public. In England, most medical students belonged to the priesthood, and in the act of snobbery, the Church had made it clear that they didn't want any senior clergy member having anything to do with surgery. A law of the Fourth Lateran Council of 1215 forbade anyone in major ecclesiastical orders from performing operations that involved making incisions. Things began to change by the mid-fifteenth century, as more laymen began graduating as surgeons.

French physician Guy de Chauliac took a different approach to invasive surgery and didn't let the Lateran Council of 1215 stop him from using a knife. He wasn't intimidated by the law, especially over a century later when he went to Bologna in 1325 to study anatomy. With his impressive reputation as a physician, he was invited to serve as a personal physician to Pope Clement VI, Pope Innocent VI (1352–1362), and Pope Urban V (1362–1370). It is said the de Chauliac may have used his surgical tools for embalming the bodies of dead popes while at his time at the Papal Court in Avignon. In 1363, de Chauliac's treatise on surgery, *Chirurgia Magna*, was completed. The seven volumes cover not only anatomy and surgery but describe surgical techniques such as intubation and tracheotomy. He truly believed that surgeons should have a clear understanding of the human body and wrote, "A surgeon who does not know his anatomy is like a blind man carving a log". His work became quite popular and was translated into several languages.

Master surgeons of English schools were content with the everyday medical theory in which animals were used for research. Anatomy was challenging to master, and students needed assistance in the way of textual commentary, diagrams, and illustrations. But these anatomical drawings were not based on direct observations of human beings; they were simply copied from existing manuscripts. Often these drawings could be in sets of five or more figures that showed veins, bones, nerves, muscles, and organs. However, these drawings looked nothing like what a surgeon would have actually seen upon entering the body. French surgeon, Henry de Mondeville (1260–1320), taught lectures using these anatomical illustrations but his student, de Chauliac, grew frustrated with this. De Chauliac felt that instead of using diagrams, it would have been more beneficial to be performing actual dissections.

In the city of Florence, surgeons could choose from a university education or a more practical, hands-on approach to learning. But to the Englishman, this was impractical. Not to say that English schools were entirely void of applied learning because they weren't. Those wishing to learn surgery studied for five or six years under a master who would support their education. As an apprentice, you had to be personable in appearance, with clean hands, keen eyesight, manual dexterity, and physical strength. During these years of apprenticeship, students would certainly learn how to perform surgical techniques and understand anatomy. And there were opportunities for dissection but perhaps not as many as one might discover in a non-English school.

The act of embalming would allow doctors to explore the inner workings of a patient and help doctors understand what caused their death. But when it came to autopsies, not too many were performed, even in cases of a violent death. In some events, such as to understand one's death and help fellow sufferers, autopsies may have been granted. But in 1299, Pope Boniface VIII (1230–1310) issued a papal bull, *Detestande Feritatis*, which was designed to prevent cruel and profane dismemberment of corpses after burial. Boniface was horrified by the practice of bodies being disembowelled and severed into pieces. It seems understandable at the time how one could see these things as an abomination towards God, but the papal bull ultimately brought the advancement of embalming to a standstill.

During the early years of the fifteenth century, foreigners began to dominate the medical practice at English courts. English students were somewhat frustrated with the faculties of medicine, such as Oxford and Cambridge, and began to look elsewhere for more in-depth education. Medical education at Italian universities was entirely different as they schooled almost all laymen. They also had more training on the workings of anatomy and surgery. Dissections took place regularly at the schools, and students could be sure to get extensive training in more invasive things. Italian students were better able to understand tumours, wounds, ulcers, dislocations, and fractures. Things were changing in other royal courts as well. In the French Court, royal surgeons in service of the House of Valois insisted on applying dry, clean dressings to a wound instead of cauterisation. But English doctors and their colleagues weren't interested and even became rude about this new approach. They chose to stick to outdated academic traditions. And so, despite this expansion of knowledge in schools across Western Europe, many English doctors still defended tradition. In 1519, Thomas Ross, Warden of the Fellowship of Surgeons in London, made it clear that surgery should only be done by those trained in manual skills, and he wasn't keen on the idea of foreigners with new ideas.

Although this archaic view of medicine seemed to infect the minds of many English surgeons, in France, Guy de Chauliac had been writing openly about different ways of preparing subjects for anatomists. It may have taken well over a century since his writings, but dissections had become part of medical education and were conducted in universities across Europe. By 1482, these dissections had finally gotten the blessing of the Pope. By 1540, things began to change in England. The newly formed Company of Barber-Surgeons of London started getting the bodies of convicted felons cut down from the gallows to practice their skills on. And they began to realize that only reading about the body was no substitute for the real thing.

If you were among the surgeons employed by royalty, you could expect that while you may be devoted to one family, your pay out would be high. Royal physicians and surgeons were sometimes paid up to £100 a year more than a non-royal physician. They were also supplied with gifts and elaborate clothing as one's appearance mattered greatly if you were treating the monarchy. John Bray (c. 1377), who was one of the royal physicians to John of Gaunt (1340–1399), as well as Edward III, was among one of the highest-paid physicians of the time, and his needs at court were well taken care of. John Arundel, Chaplain (d. 1477) and physician to King Henry VI in 1454, was given enormous royal advancements, including seven rectories and he was named Bishop of Chichester in 1459. His wife and son also enjoyed the royal luxuries bestowed upon him. Henry VI was also extremely generous to his physician John Somerset (d. 1454), allowing him to exchange his fees for an elaborate life estate.

When one pictures medicine in the Middle Ages, the image of the unkempt barber-surgeon comes to mind. With blood smeared about their apron, the barber-surgeon could give you a close shave or pull your rotting teeth out. The image of this medieval man with a host of tools that would give anyone nightmares probably wasn't far off. Barber-surgeons were laymen, who despite their lack of a medical degree, could be pretty useful in minor surgical procedures. The Middle Ages gives us a much more brutal and crude way of dealing with illness for sure, and the iconic barber-surgeon was a familiar medical practitioner. They could be tasked with bloodletting, amputation, setting dislocated limbs, lancing boils, or suturing wounds. Although authorities felt that barber-surgeons were little more than butchers, they did have their place in medieval society.

The role of barber-surgeons and physicians were almost entirely separated. While the physician saw to the upper class, residing at court, the barber-surgeons often catered to a lower class of people. And because physicians felt that the act of surgery was often beneath their dignity, this left plenty of work for barber-surgeons. The working class of peasants and craftsmen allowed the barber-surgeons to really get their hands dirty. Barber-surgeons were there to pick up the pieces of what tasks physicians just wouldn't do. They indeed arose as a common type of surgeon, who may have lacked the education and high regard of an actual surgeon. Their tasks were often messy and less desirable, but over time the barber-surgeons were able to become more independent and claim more of a name for themselves.

One of the earliest roles of the barber-surgeon was at the monastery. They were employed around Europe because of their skill as a barber. Monks, whose hair was tonsured regularly, needed to have someone on hand to perform this religious practice. As time went on, barbers were allowed to do more than just cut hair at a monastery. As monasteries began taking on the role of a hospital and healing sanctuary, the job of the barber-surgeon changed as well. They took on the more medical tasks of bloodletting or setting limbs.

Barber-surgeons took advantage of the thirteenth-century law passed in France, which required all physicians in training to swear not to perform surgery. This left a lot of opportunity for barber-surgeons to take up the needs of patients that physicians would not fulfil. Aside from bloodletting, barber-surgeons grew quite experienced at amputation. While a lot of this was practised in war, several common afflictions would call for the need for amputation. With no way to prevent infection, diseased limbs were a common and excruciating thing. Using a special curved knife, a barber-surgeon could cut through all flesh and muscle quickly and saw through the bone. All of this was done with no anaesthetic, of course. Trepanation, a procedure common during the later Middle Ages into the

Renaissance, was another task that barber-surgeons became familiar with. By boring a hole into the skull of the afflicted patient, it was believed that trepanation would relieve pressure on the brain, as well as cure seizures or behavioural problems. Drilling a hole in one's head would have allowed demons or evil forces to escape.

After long periods of training and apprenticeship, a young barber-surgeon might eventually want to go into business for himself. From the fourteenth century onwards, a license was needed for this. The guild would protect a barber-surgeon but the right to having a permit remained controversial throughout the Middle Ages because of the growing rivalry between barber-surgeons and physicians. Physicians most likely had within their grasp, a decent selection of medical books on disease and surgery. And although barbers probably didn't accumulate as many, they still wanted to learn to master Galenic medicine. Because of the growing need for bloodletting and minor operations, especially after the twelfth century, most barber-surgeons were able to make something of themselves. This was the case even with the arrogant attitude of physicians and royal surgeons, who thought of themselves as being above all others. But it wasn't entirely easy for barber-surgeons to make their way in society. In 1307, in London, barber-surgeons were warned that their advertising was too brutal, for in their shop windows they often displayed human bowels or vats of blood which was extremely unsettling to the public. They were often looked down upon for working on the Sabbath and became the subject of malpractice lawsuits. However, in Paris in 1493, physicians slowly began to permit barbers access to better medical training, and this infuriated surgeons. Still, some London surgeons did begin to employ the barbers as assistants, but by no means were they their professional equal.

In 1423, plans for a joint college began to unfold, but it was expected that barber-surgeons would take direction from their professional superiors. Even though this collaboration was unthinkable to the upper elite, they did eventually compromise and learn to work together. In English towns, the role of the barber-surgeon was slowly becoming more accepted. Between 1450 and 1499, there was a need for more practitioners in York and Canterbury due to the number of sick pilgrims that were going to the cathedrals.

By the mid-1500s, barber-surgeons were able to pass through ports to perform their trade, but the town ordinances still had them work openly in shops so that authorities would be able to keep a better eye on them. While some barber-surgeons may have wanted to escape the watchful eye of the guild, most probably paid for their short term permits to practice.

Physicians, surgeons, and barber-surgeons faced everyday dangers in the simplest of operations or unpredictable effects of medications. They always faced the risk of being sued. Patients often sued simply because they couldn't afford to pay the bill. Some doctors would take payment in the form of bonds and securities to ensure some future financial closure. And many medieval doctors did have a great concern for the poor and would cut their fees or give free service as a form of charity. In fifteenth century France, highly qualified doctors and surgeons were called on to serve the community as an act of public health. This service was especially prevalent during epidemics. Often, they were paid by the city or by lords for their service to the community. It was looked at as a duty to God to tend to the poor.

The apothecary was the one who prepared and sold medicines and drugs. In the Middle Ages, this was exactly right. The apothecary was a medieval pharmacist and was relied on heavily by not only the physicians but laymen as well. The history of the apothecary as a profession dates back to 2600 BCE during ancient Babylon. Throughout time, due to the knowledge of Islamic pharmacists during the Islamic Golden Age, Arabs became some of the most significant contributors to Greek pharmaceuticals. Developments in the Arab world spread into Europe as many suppliers of medicine came from overseas. Arab pharmacists were responsible for mixing sugar along with many medications to make them more palatable, often taking Greek recipes and mixing them with sweet syrup or powder. Electuaries, which was often the name for the thick, soft, confections of herbs and spices, became common in aiding digestion. Arab writer Masawaih Al-Mardini, of the eleventh century, was hailed in the west as "the evangelist of pharmacy". He devoted twelve chapters of a text known as, *The Grabadbin* to the production of electuaries. Apothecaries widely used his text in Western Europe. Apothecaries had initially been part of the grocer business in the western world but began to join with physicians to supply drugs. They often trained through apprenticeships and, starting in the 1500s, began to get some formal education at universities.

An apothecary could make recipes depending on the wealth of their customer, the prescription, and what was available at the time.

Apothecaries serving the royal court could be assured more access to supplies as they were often ordered in bulk. For the layperson and those lower on the social ladder, one would turn to the marketplaces for their supplies. But it was the goods coming from the East Indies, Persia, and Egypt that made up the majority of things used in medicines. The market in the west in regard to foreign imports was always limitless. Often a monastery would have an attending apothecary on staff just for making and dispensing medications.

One of the most celebrated drugs for sale in medieval Europe was something called theriac, which was believed to have limited medicinal powers. Theriac was a concoction initially formulated by the Greeks in the first century and spread to the ancient worlds of Persia, China, and India through trade. Theriac could prevent swelling, help to alleviate a blocked intestine, get rid of pustules, restore lost speech, remove a dead child from the womb, heal wounds and bites, help with a prolapsed uterus and protect against the plague. There didn't seem to be anything this medication couldn't do. Henry of Grosmont, 1st Duke of Lancaster (1310–1361), mentioned it in literature as part of a cure of the soul, but this cure was also "made of poison to destroy another poison". Grosmont also thought that theriac was part of moral curative. Since God had sent the Black Death as punishment, theriac was an appropriate remedy. Because theriac frequently contained opium, it did have a soothing effect against pain. Part of its appeal was that it was a costly import, and westerners thought that anything foreign was like liquid gold. The ancient Greeks had produced a variety of theriacs as antidotes to snake bites. The history of theriac begins with King Mithridates VI of Pontus (135 BCE–63 BCE), who experimented with poisons and antidotes on his prisoners. These experiments eventually led him to claim that he had discovered a remedy for every poisonous substance. He mixed all of his successful antidotes into a single one, called *mithridatium*. Mithridatium contained opium, myrrh, saffron, ginger, cinnamon, and castor, along with forty other ingredients. As his medical notes made their way into Roman hands, they improved upon them, bringing the total number of components to sixty-four. Although it was supposed to combat the effects of poison, it was more of a poison itself. Galen prescribed theriac for many different things, and it took him close to a month to make it. On top of the length of time it took to make, it was thought that theriac should be left to mature for years by the process of fermentation. Galen also devoted an entire book to it, entitled *Theriake*. Physicians and apothecaries learned of theriac from classical and Arab sources, the most influential being *Tractatus de Tyriaca*, which was a thirteenth-century translation of Averroes. Before his death of the plague in 1348, physician Gentile da Foligno recommended that to be effective, theriac should be aged at least one year. It was also believed to be safer if children didn't ingest it but instead rub it on as a salve

Theriac was used not only as an antidote but as a way to eliminate phlegmatic and melancholy humours. It was expensive, complicated, and time-consuming to make, as well as dangerous. Apothecaries in Venice had strict guidelines in 1268 for preparing it. Those who imported it into England were held responsible for its quality. Authorities began to inspect it as it came into English ports. It was essential to make sure that it was pure and not mixed with salt or rice in the hopes of scamming both doctor and patient.

France introduced stiff regulations on apothecaries and insisted on a level of training and supervision of staff, as well as uniform standards of weights and measurements. In England, there weren't very rigid systems for training and licensing, but they at least had to obey the correct use of weights and measurements. There seemed to be some question as to whether drugs and spices should be weighed before or after being cleaned of impurities as this would alter their weight. There was also some dispute over who should be stamping bundles as they came into port cities.

At the close of the thirteenth century, London apothecaries began to form their own kind of guild to uphold standards and to protect their traders. In 1340, they merged with spicers and grocers, forming one stable organization that led to improvements. In 1417, the government began to conduct inspections on goods, and in 1540, the London College of Physicians began to regulate the drug trade against counterfeit and other abuses.

Like royal physicians and surgeons, apothecaries who were employed by the monarchy were paid very well. King Edward III gave sixpence a day for life to Coursus de Gangeland, the apothecary of London. Edward was thankful for the services bestowed upon him while he was sick in Scotland during 1345. Also, in Scotland, John the Apothecary was given generous payment for materials used to embalm Robert the Bruce in 1329. John Gryce, Sergeant of the Confectionary to Henry VII, was awarded a tenement house for his services. Henry's frugalness made him cautious in the matter of gifts. But the more generous King Henry VI offered his apothecaries very lavish payments. He lined the pockets of his apothecary, Richard Hakedy, giving him a life's pension as well as the title of King's Esquire. Hakedy was very involved in the treatment of the king when Henry fell ill in 1454. He was instructed by the king's doctors to supply the following: electuaries, potions, syrups, confections, laxatives, clysters, suppositories, cataplasms, gargles, and baths. The royal apothecary was responsible for perfuming and fumigating the royals' clothes and bedding, as well as making up preparations for prescriptions by doctors.

King Henry VIII was, in his own right, an apothecary, although not formally trained. Much like his father, Henry had always had a keen interest in medicine. Amateur though he was, he found the preparation and compounding of plasters and ointments exhilarating. He kept a royal collection of 114 favourite recipes for "plasters, cataplasms, balms, waters, lotions and decorations", thirty-two of these were devised by the King himself. Many of the remedies made by Henry must have been for his personal use. He already had an irrational fear of getting sick and had been known to lock himself away during outbreaks of sweating sickness or other ailments. And so, having his own go-to pharmacy must have brought him some comfort. The king had an ulcerous sore on his leg that had begun to plague him even early on in his reign and was known for experimenting with several homemade plasters to ease his pain and cool the inflammation. Henry had an insatiable lust for sexual endeavours, and it seems it may have brought its own host of problems. The "King's Grace's Ointment" was concocted to "cool and dry and comfort the Member" and another ointment to "dry excoriations and comfort the Member". It doesn't take much imagination to figure out that Henry's appetite for pleasing the ladies of the court probably left him somewhat chafed. It might explain Henry's need to use plenty of oil of roses and rose water for its sweet smell. A young monarch could use whatever means necessary to boost his pheromones. The king used ingredients that were known for their cooling, healing, and softening properties, such as fenugreek and linseed. He used lead and turpentine for his plasters and more exotic ingredients like powdered red coral. Henry also employed his own royal apothecaries and paid them quite well. Richard Babham was the king's apothecary for most of his life and was paid accordingly. Cuthbert Blackden, another of the king's apothecaries, tended to Princess Mary as well and was awarded some of Queen Jane's jewellery when she passed away. Thomas Alsop was Henry's apothecary in his later years, as well as through the reign of King Edward and Queen Mary, the king's children. Alsop was there as Henry's health declined and crafted the king his glasses as he aged. He was also responsible for making potpourri for the king's coffin when he died.

As the reign of Henry VIII went on, people dabbling in herbal remedies started to create competition with the physicians. Many English apothecaries stated that they knew as much about compounding medicine as any physician, and they were probably right. To men like Thomas Linacre (1460–1524), Henry's personal physician, it seemed mad that anyone less trained dare to think of themselves as a healer. But as the population of England grew, so did the ranks of skilled or semi-skilled practitioners, whether they called themselves barber-surgeons or apothecaries or even physicians. There became an obvious need for supervision and control over this mass of practitioners, which began to consist of more and more fraudulent people. It was with the full backing of the king in 1512, that physicians pressed for legislation that gave them authority to deal with the problem. Parliament passed the first in a series of acts that dealt chiefly with London. These acts restricted the practice of medicine within a seven-mile radius of the city unless the Bishop of London had licensed the practitioner. In the 1540s, two more laws were passed, which reconfirmed the authority of the physicians, giving them complete control over both barber-surgeons and apothecaries.

The first dental school wasn't started until the mid-1800s in the United States, but that doesn't mean that practitioners in the Middle Ages didn't treat their fair share of tooth problems. Care of the teeth was mostly limited to non-invasive treatment but works citing dentistry are quite plentiful. Favourite cures were herbal and also included prayer and charms. And depending on the practitioner, treatment could be influenced by the presentation of the humours.

One of the earliest texts that support the care of the mouth is the *Chirurgia of Roger Frugard* (1140–1195) that was written in northern Italy. He recognised cancer of the mouth if the flesh was blackened and hard. He believed that in the acute stages of the disease, you could cut into the healthy tissue surrounding the cancer, cauterise the wound and then seal it with egg yolk. After three days, the mouth should be rinsed with wine, and then a lotion applied made from wine and honey, honeysuckle, and pomegranate. Frugard advocated for the placement of a dental tent in the case of an open fracture. The patient should eat soft foods and anoint the wound with powder. For pain in the teeth and the gums, he advised that the patient should inhale smoke through a funnel made from henbane and leek seeds over hot coals.

In the small village of Myddfai, Wales, a collection of remedies was put together in the early thirteenth century. Toothache was a common complaint and could be treated with herbal remedies. The roots of pellitory of Spain should be shaped into balls and then retained between the cheek and bothersome tooth:

> as long as you walk a mile with moderate steps, and as the saliva collects, spit it away. When you think that the ball had been there as long as that, put in another and walk backwards and forwards for the same space of time; after that put in the third, then lie in bed, and warm yourself well, and when you have slept you will be free from pain. This I have proved and found to be a present remedy for toothache.

It was also recommended that you could prevent toothache by "whenever you wash, rub the inside of your ears with your fingers".

It was believed by many practitioners, since Anglo Saxon times, that a worm was the cause of your trouble when you were inflicted with oral pain. Patients were sometimes accused of swallowing a worm, and one of the Welsh cures against this said tooth worm were as follows:

> Take a candle of sheep suet, some eryngo seed being mixed therewith, and burn it as near the tooth as possible, some cold water being held under the candle. The worms will drop into the water to escape the heat of the candle.

Several recipes to aid in painless extraction called for varying ingredients to be made into a powder, like "Seek some ants with their eggs and powder, have this powder blown into the tooth through a quill, and be careful that it does not touch another tooth".

This paste was to be placed in a cavity if an extraction was needed, with the reminder that it did not touch another tooth. "Insert the paste in the tooth so as to fill the cavity. It will cause the tooth to fall from your jaw but have a care that it does not touch another tooth".

Physician Gilbertus Anglicus (1180–1250) made several references to tooth care in his *Compendium*, a collection of medical recipes grouped by the area of the body they were aimed to treat. The cause of "stinking of the mouth" or bad breath were caused by corruption of the teeth and gums, stomach problems, or lung disorders. He advised that in the case of a problem with the teeth and gums, any rotten flesh should be removed, and the patient was to gargle with birch and mint soaked in wine. The gums should then be rubbed with a rough linen cloth until they bled. And the patient was to chew marjoram oregano, mint, and pellitory then. Anglicus also wrote on toothache, worms, and rotting of the teeth. He believed that these were caused mainly by the imbalance of the humours. Eating hot or cold food in quick succession or overheating of the head could cause the cheeks to be swollen and red. Coldness of the humours caused the cheeks to be pale and teeth to be cold. Moisture could cause the cheeks to be swollen and soft, dryness caused hardness but little swelling. Phlegm caused pallor of the cheeks, and melancholy caused yellow discolouration of the cheeks. Anglicus's treatment varied depending on the cause of the toothache. Bloodletting was advised in several cases, but if excessive coldness was the culprit, then it was important not to bleed the patient but repeatedly place and remove a cup from the neck. Toothache could also be relieved by inhaling smoke from burnt, wet rose petals. If stomach problems were the cause of your pain, you used an ointment of mastic, clay mixed with iron oxide, dried juice of the dragon's blood tree, all mixed with egg whites, placed directly on the temples. Worms in the teeth can be overcome by inhaling the smoke from hot henbane. If the pain caused by worms was because of excessive blood, you could simply be bled. For pain caused by extreme cold, marjoram mixed with horsemint and wine could be gargled or applied as a poultice with honey or salt to the gums. However, Anglicus readily admitted in his text that all of the treatments could very well fail. He advocated opiates being administered, and if that failed, the tooth should be extracted.

Theodoric (1205–1296), a surgeon from northern Italy, referred to fractures of the jaw in his Chirurgia. His works include descriptions of suturing and splinting as well.

> A fracture of the mandible or maxilla, or of some other part of the face, if associated with cuts or abrasions, should, after the wound has been thoroughly cleansed, have the lips of the wound brought together as perfectly as the ingenuity of the physician can devise; and the separated portions of the skin and flesh should be rejoined as accurately as they were in the healthy state; and, if it should be necessary, according to the size of the wound, let it be sutured. And after applying a little bolstering pad, according to previous teaching, bind it up skillfully.

Theodoric believed that if a fracture were bandaged correctly, it would heal correctly. He believed in leaving the bandage in place for ten days and rebound if the patient was in too much pain. The patient should then be kept quiet and calm and given only liquid foods, and after twenty days, he should be healed.

John of Gaddesden had a different approach when it came to dentistry. His works contained much on charms, sympathetic medicine, and folklore. Although his work became very popular, it was not so well received by his colleague, Guy de Chauliac. De Chauliac stated that "it was a stupid rehash of the worst of medical lore".

Gaddesden stood firm that one could dislocate their jaw by merely yawning. He says it was a rare incident, but nonetheless, provided the following method of treatment:

> an assistant should hold the patient's head while the surgeons puts his thumb into the mouth, and after moving the jaw from side to side, he must extend it suddenly until the upper and lower teeth are on a level, then let him reduce it. Another method, which is successful if carried out as soon as the dislocation has happened, is for the patient to give himself a sharp blow on the chin, in a backward and at the same time upward direction. A friend who is present may be asked to do this.

He was sure that sudden death could be caused by yawning and he was convinced that evil spirits might be able to enter the body through the open mouth.

Guy de Chauliac pointed out that problems of the teeth should be dealt with by the barber-surgeon and not the doctor. De Chauliac referred to the use of dental tools when performing an extraction. He spoke of the following instruments for assisting the patient; razors, spatulas, straight and curved pliers, probes, and curettage knives. He thought that loose teeth should be secured with a gold wire. But if they were to fall out, false teeth could be made. He stated that the replacement teeth could be made from human teeth or teeth made from the bone of a cow.

As we look back on the writings of medical practitioners, we should stop and think of how different the world was. While the teachings seem barbaric and downright cruel, we have to tell ourselves that this was between five and eight hundred years ago. Cutting someone open to have them bleed out deliberately seems absurd to us now, but that was the believed method of the time. Forcing a hot iron into an already angry wound makes us cringe to think of it, but in the mind of the medieval surgeon, he was doing you a favour. As I have mentioned earlier, I genuinely believe that physicians of the time took the Hippocratic Oath seriously and thought that they were not harming their patients but helping them to the best of their ability.

Chapter Seven

Medicine on the Battlefield

Many of the advancements in surgery and treatment have to be attributed to learning while on the battlefield. The medieval world at war was something none of us can comprehend. Casual violence in the Middle Ages was so high that even doctors who weren't trained in combat got experience with head wounds and internal injuries. But to be a practitioner on the battlefield would have been an eye-opening experience. For as long as war has existed between man, the battlefield has been an opportunity not only to observe injury but to treat it. The techniques used by surgeons were some of the boldest innovations to date, as so many of them had never been used before. The relationship that has always existed between medicine and war fully embraces the outward displays of two of the most primitive humanities. The most basic of these principles derive from the very beginning of man's existence, self-preservation through aggression. The warrior's intuition is to destroy while the healer's is to heal. The very challenge of medicine at war was to unravel the dire consequences that man's folly has always committed onto one another.

The Greek word by which Hippocrates referred to a healer was *Iatros*, which means *extractor of arrows*. Ironically, the very thing that ultimately destroyed the Golden Age of Greece was a contagious bacteria or plague that infected the Greek troops with a vengeance. Until the understanding of proper cleanliness, the dangers of encampment lay in the basics of sanitation being of little interest to commanders. And as history has taught us, this neglect would wipe out an entire fleet of battle-hardened soldiers, no matter how tough they were.

During the Battle of Agincourt, the English army already had a disadvantage as the fearless French warriors outnumbered them three to one. And when dysentery began to spread through Henry V's army, it only made their thirteen-mile journey to Calais worse. The intestinal inflammation and frequent, uncontrollable diarrhoea would wipe out a quarter of the English army. Not only was there fever and fatigue, but the constant looseness of bowels posed a considerable problem. Military camps were hotbeds for communicable diseases. Often, illness killed more soldiers than the actual battle itself. Easily transmittable and usually fatal, dysentery could decimate an army. Because doctors believed that diseases were brought on by an imbalance of the four humours, the idea of contagious disease was not clearly understood. Because there were no sanitation standards, soldiers had always been in the habit of relieving themselves wherever they saw fit. Agincourt took place in what was already muddy ground so the bathroom habits of soldiers quickly turned encampments into soiled breeding grounds for what they called the Bloody Flux. Because of their lax attitudes and lack of understanding of sanitation and personal hygiene, soldiers quickly spread the disease among their fellow comrades. They didn't see it necessary to wash their hands, and in the heat of battle, it's understandable that this was their last priority. Human waste likely contaminated any clean water available to them. Henry's men were sick and starving by the time they reached Calais, and yet despite having nothing in their favour, they still defeated the French army.

When French King Charles VIII invaded Naples in the first of the Italian Wars, he didn't expect that a painful and repulsive plague would spread throughout his men at a ferocious rate. In the summer of 1494, 50,000 French soldiers headed to Northern Italy to claim the kingdom of Naples as a base to launch a campaign to the Crusades. By February 1495, they were victorious in their efforts, and the French soldiers found reason to celebrate. They drank and self-indulged themselves in illicit sex. After only a short amount of time, Charles' soldiers began to notice that something was terribly wrong. Genital ulcers, fever, and aches began to trouble the men. These symptoms were soon followed by painful, pus-filled abscesses that smelled putrid. The sores spread over their entire bodies. The French soldiers had contracted syphilis. The army began to get so ill that they had to retreat to France. This caused the disease to spread throughout France, into Switzerland and Germany, and by the year 1497, it had spread to England and Scotland, continuing its vicious sweep throughout much of Europe.

In the early days of the Roman Empire, the Roman's considered medicine to be too "Greek". Therefore, it was suspect and domesticated soldiers who brought their own bandages to care for themselves and each other. But by 200 BCE, medical care had advanced, and the designation of wound surgeons in an army began to take place. However, it was not until the reign of Julius Caesar that the Roman military medical system began to form. Better care for soldiers was offered, along with well-equipped hospitals and treatment centres. Unfortunately, with the fall of the Roman Empire, all of these miraculous advancements in battlefield medicine disappeared from the west.

While nobles went to war with their own surgeons during the Middle Ages, the simple soldier went without. Medical care was rarely offered unless, of course, one provided it for themselves. Ordinary soldiers died quickly, or if they didn't right away, they would most likely succumb to the wrath of the enemy while laying hurt on the battlefield. During the Crusades, no method of caring for the sick and wounded soldiers had been organised. They were subject to the horrific blows of swords and battle axes that created ghastly wounds. Even the noble knight, with better access to a physician, did not fare much better. American medical historian and Colonel, Fielding Garrison (1870–1935) created a very vivid description of a wounded knight from a group of medieval epics.

> We see the wounded knight laid upon the ground, his wounds examined, washed and bandaged, often with a wimple from a woman's forehead; the various practices of giving a stimulating wound-drink to relieve faintness, or pouring oil or wine into wounds, of stanching haemorrhage or relieving pain by sundry herbs, of wound sucking to prevent internal haemorrhage, the mumbling of charms over wounds; the many balsams, salves, and plasters used in wound-dressing; the feeling of the pulse in the cephalic, median and hepatic veins to ascertain the patient's chances of recovery; the danger of suffocation or heat stroke from the heavy visored helmet and coat of mail; the eventual transportation of the patient by hand, on shields or litters, on horseback or on litters attached to horses; the sumptuous chambers and couches reserved for the high-born, and the calling of physicians, usually from the famous schools of Salerno or Montpellier, in grave cases. The ministrations of womankind are always depicted with great charm and prelude the organization of sick nursing in the later medieval period.

And still, despite all futile attempts to save the life of a wounded knight, in most cases, battlefield injuries proved deadly.

The weapons of an English medieval knight in combat were something to be impressed with, even in the days of modern warfare. The long sword, wooden lance with an iron tip metal-headed mace, battle-axe, and dagger could inflict fatal injuries, even on an opponent in full armour. The image of a knight, mounted on horseback, wielding a lance was a terrifying sight. However, a dismounted one with a sword that could sever limbs was a weapon in itself. Even if a knight was robbed of his sword, he had been trained to kill with an axe, mace, or dagger. The years of gruelling training the medieval knight endured made him the ultimate killing machine.

A knight's most important weapon was his sword. Blessed by a priest, a knight's sword was the weapon most likely used to give him his status from the beginning. Swords were lethal weapons, long, heavy, and sharp, and designed to remove a limb in one fell swoop. The medieval longsword used by a knight could have varying degrees of dimensions, but all were meant to thrust, cut, and kill. Double-edged swords could be as long as forty inches in length and were designed to be swung using both hands on the grip. The tapering could differ slightly on a sword; it could be more pronounced at the end and widen somewhat towards the handle. A shorter, wide-bladed sword would have been used primarily for slashing at your opponent. In use since 1280 CE, a blade with a flattened cross-section was designed to pierce plate armour. The Falchion sword, developed in thirteenth century France, had a short, broad curved blade, sometimes with one edge curved and the other straight. These weapons were specially weighted towards the tip, which made them first-rate in chopping off an extremity. Along with a sword, most knights carried a dagger, which was a miniature version of the longsword with only one sharpened edge.

The medieval joust was the perfect place for a knight to practice his skills needed to stay alive on the battlefield. A knight had to be skilled at guiding his horse while carrying a lance in one hand and in the other a shield. All the while keeping his balance in the saddle and successfully striking a moving target. A knight's lance could be as long as 10 ft in length. They were usually made from ash or cypress, with a steel tip at the end.

Popular in Europe during the twelfth century, the mace was a shaft made of wood with a head of copper, with protruding, rounded projections or flanges. Some versions had a spiked ball known as a morning star that was usually made of steel or iron. To be sure that a mace was not lost after a blow, a strap was worn about the knight's wrist and attached to the base of the shaft.

The medieval axe either had a widening blade and long shaft or a thinner, more pointed blade and short shaft. The Poleaxe was a combination of a hammer and axe with a spike. The Ravensbill, the Halberd, and the Glaive were other variations of a knight's axe, and their use often depended on whether the warrior was on horseback or on foot.

One of the most notorious points in history tells us just how deadly these weapons, as well as the medieval knight, really were. The Battle of Bosworth, fought on 22 August 1485, would change English history forever. Bosworth was the last battle of the War of the Roses, a series of English wars fought for control of the throne. Lancastrian Henry Tudor and his army of supporters would defeat the Yorkist king, Richard III, and seize the crown, marking the beginning of the Tudor dynasty. But King Richard didn't go down without a fight. The thirty-two-year-old king succumbed to Henry's forces and was surrounded before being stabbed to death. Researchers at the University of Leicester were able to piece together how he died after his remains were found in a Leicester parking lot in 2012.

Through much analysis, professionals believe that Richard sustained nine injuries to his head and one to his pelvis. His skeletal remains show that he received blows by a dagger to his cranium, cheekbones, jaw, and tenth rib. The king had most likely removed his helmet, or it had fallen off in battle. His head wounds show that there was no protection and he had most likely been on his knees when the fatal blows to the back of his head were delivered. It was believed that Richard had dismounted his horse in an attempt to save his throne through hand-to-hand combat. There were no consistent wounds on his arms which leads researchers to believe that the rest of his body, sans his head, was still covered in heavy armour. Guy Rutty, professor at the University of Leicester pathology unit, says:

> The most likely injuries to have caused the king's death are the two of the inferior aspect of the skull – a large sharp force trauma, possibly from a sword or staff weapon, such as a halberd or bill,

and a penetrating injury from the tip of an edged weapon. Richard's head injuries are consistent with some near-contemporary accounts of battle, which suggest that Richard abandoned his horse after it became stuck in a mire and was killed while fighting his enemies.

Richard was stabbed repeatedly once he was surrounded and several of those blows likely came after his death. His crown was pulled from his head and placed on the head of his Lancastrian enemy, declaring a new king of England.

This new king of England brought something else with him to the Battle of Bosworth as well; the Sweating Sickness. The English Sweat is deeply engrained in the history of the country, and researchers are reasonably confident that it was the new Tudor king who was responsible for the outbreak. French soldiers, who were helping to support Henry Tudor's claim to the throne, may have brought it with them to the battlefield. Lord Stanley, 1st Earl of Derby (1435–1504), claimed it was the sweating sickness that caused him to withdraw his army and side with Henry Tudor. And the disease followed the new king and his men back to London, where it killed around 15,000 people in six weeks. It is thought the French who supported Henry Tudor picked up the disease during their campaign against the Ottoman Empire in 1480, and unknowingly brought it to England.

It was evident that there was nothing that could have been done to save Richard at the time of his defeat. Sweating Sickness or not, even in modern times, the blows delivered by medieval weapons would have proved impressive to surgeons. But that didn't mean that wound care was unsophisticated in the Middle Ages. Anything that broke through the skin or caused lacerations threatened the inner workings of the body. Wounds not only penetrated but introduced bacteria and infection. However, medieval surgeons on the battlefield still tried to heal even the worst injuries if they thought there was a chance. The body could be wounded, but it could also be put back together. It could be healed with ointments, honey, sutures, plasters, and bandages. In the world of medieval warfare, healing wounds was just as significant a part of everyday life as inflicting them was. Soldiers certainly understood that physical wounds needed to be treated hastily. They should have been easily and successfully treated, but instead, many turned gangrenous, painful, and eventually fatal. But not all wounds led to infection and death and it was the battle surgeon that went above and beyond to utilise their skills. Many misconceptions suggest that medicine during the Middle Ages was wholly backward and primitive. And while it may have been primitive when compared to the advancements of the Romans, medieval medicine on the battlefield did evolve over time.

Honey had been used by the ancient Egyptians as a wound treatment as early as 3000 BCE. It was an integral part of their wound care in that it included washing the wound, applying a plaster that was made from honey, animal fat, and vegetable fibre, and utilizing a clean bandage to the injury. Through time medieval people also grew aware of the beneficial properties of honey. It made an excellent disinfectant and antimicrobial agent. There is evidence that honey was kept, probably by the apothecary, in large stores in medieval castles to use for its medicinal properties. Honey was a vital resource during warfare and was used by medieval surgeons.

The use of maggots to clear necrotised skin was something that had been discovered centuries ago. Military physicians around the time of the Renaissance state that soldiers whose wounds had become colonised with maggots experienced less morbidity than soldiers whose injuries had not been inhabited by them. Although the thought of fly larva is somewhat revolting to patients and probably their caregivers as well, maggots hold an exceptional place in the history of wound care. French surgeon Ambroise Pare (1510–1590) realised that maggot infected patients recovered much quicker than others. We aren't sure if he attributed this quick recovery to the maggots per se. Pare believed that the fly larva was a natural part of the putrefaction process of dead tissue. However, for the most part, due to the fall of the Roman Empire, wound care in the Middle Ages regressed to potions and charms.

In the event of an artery being severed, battle surgeons would treat them with finger pressure or by twisting the artery into submission with hooks. Attempts to tie them off with stout thread would sometimes be successful but often resulted in infection and haemorrhaging despite a surgeon's best efforts. A cauterising iron may have been applied to bleeding tissue, usually doing more to destroy the very flesh the practitioner was desperate to save.

The Battle of Crecy on 26 August 1346 may have established the effectiveness of the longbow on the battlefield, but it also gave surgeons something new to think about. They now had to consider the effect of gunshot wounds as King Edward III's English army was equipped with several types of gunpowder weapons. This presented a new challenge for the surgeons tending to the wounded Frenchman. While the blade of a knife cut cleanly, bullets veered off into all directions after entering the body. The English army had already burnt a path of destruction throughout France, sacking many towns on the way to Paris. King Philips VI's army's attacks were broken up by the active fire from English archers, and when it came down to hand to hand combat, it was described as "murderous, without pity, cruel and very horrible".

And on top of that, doctors discovered that the bullet could rip its way through tissue, introducing infection into the wounds. Doctors were convinced that bullets must be made with poison. The methods devised for removing the poison were by debridement, the act of cutting away injured or destroyed tissue. Surgeons used forceps to remove bullets, as well as other bits of matter that had made its way into the wound. It was thought that pouring hot oil or grease into the bullet hole would ensure a secure method to remove the bullet. Over one hundred years later, German doctor Hieronymus Brunschwig (1450–1512) would elaborate on the theory in 1497. Recognised for his treatment of gunshot wounds, he recommended pouring bacon fat into the opening to encourage pus to loosen the impacted object and help lubricate its exit.

Giovanni da Vigo (1450–1525), Italian surgeon to Pope Julius II (1443–1513), published a book on surgery in 1514, called *Practica in are chirurgica copiosa*. His book was composed of nine books on anatomy, ulcers, wounds, and fractures. Da Vigo's book is also one of the earliest discussing the treatment of gunshot wounds. Like surgeons before his time, he also believed that gunpowder was poison and that boiling oil should be poured into the wound. Although today we know that such treatment of gunshot wounds is not sufficient, da Vigo's book on surgery was quite successful. It was translated into English, Latin, Italian, and French and was used into the seventeenth century as a reference.

It was from da Vigo and Brunschwig that French surgeon Ambroise Pare learned. The young barber-surgeon served four monarchs and was a pioneer in battlefield medicine. Most importantly, in the treatment of wounds. Pare was also known for preparing scalding hot oil to pour into missile wounds. A procedure, he "found the most miserable, and pernicious kind of invention ... this hellish engine, tempered by the malice and guidance of man". Although many of Pare's innovations followed the Renaissance, I feel it is important to mention him because he clearly showed enormous compassion on the battlefield. He may have learned the technique of pouring hot oil into a gunshot wound, but Pare was also a profound observer. After practising the hot oil method after learning about it, he was able to form his own thoughts and variations on the procedure. The hellish procedure Pare described left soldiers in absolute agony. He was able to understand that besides the searing pain a soldier would endure, that the treatment wasn't overly effective. Soldiers that had instead been treated with an ointment containing turpentine recovered more effectively. Turpentine had been used medicinally by Ferdinand Magellan at the beginning of the 1500s. Pare changed battlefield history in the way that he avoided cauterisation after that and published his first book in 1545 on the method of treating wounds.

The Battle of Hastings in 1066 is the battle that defined England. William, Duke of Normandy, had his sights set on invading England for some time. Harold II, King of England (1022–1066), sat on the throne. Harold was an earl and a member of the Anglo-Saxons. The Saxons had established themselves in Great Britain since the fifth century. They were a group of fierce warriors with the very best armour, and they carried the infamous battle-axe, their weapon of choice. William had laid claim to the throne after Edward the Confessor (1003–1066), the last King of the Anglo-Saxons, had died. A distant cousin of Edward's, William claimed that Edward had promised him the English throne while visiting France in 1051. On the morning of 14 October 1066, William began his invasion of England along the coast of Normandy. His troops were exhausted but he attacked nonetheless. The battle began just after dawn and would rage for nine long hours. At sunset that same day, Harold II would be defeated, and his Anglo-Saxon forces would disassemble. William's army of archers, soldiers, and mounted knights would prove to be too fierce, even for the hardened military wielding battle axes. The English army had been better suited, with heavy armour that absorbed missiles and spurs thrust from the enemy's infantry. But there was, however, a "chink" in the armour. The area of the eyes that sat below the helmet or behind the eye slits was an open target for a crafty archer. The English king sat tall in his saddle and attracted the attention of many archers. In the heat of battle, he had been hit in his right eye before being pulled from his horse by William's men.

Perhaps the best description we have of the incident lies in the Bayeux Tapestry, a 230-foot-long embroidered piece of linen that was made after the Battle of Hastings. Among many other drawings of battle scenes, the tapestry details how Harold pulled the arrow from his eye. He most likely pulled the arrow out before collapsing and falling from his horse. Historians believe that the arrow struck near his eye but possibly missed the eyeball itself. The arrow most likely funnelled itself in through Harold's orbital apex and into the sinuses, where it hit an artery. It may have entered the brain but as he pulled it out, he likely caused extensive bleeding as well. Harold was knocked to the ground wearing over 100lbs of thick, cumbersome armour. The weight of his protection would have prevented him from getting back up again.

The Bayeux Tapestry then shows knights attacking Harold from many different directions. William's men hacked away at his torso and limbs until he was dismembered. Hopefully, for his sake, this mutilation took place after Harold died. Sources tell us that he most likely had already gone before being attacked. Injuries were plentiful on both sides, from mounted knights, the Saxon battle-axe, and the Norman arrow barrage. But on the evening of 14 October, the headless bodies were cleared from the field. A tent was pitched, and William, along with his blood-covered filthy men, celebrated their victory with a dinner. William was crowned King of England on Christmas Day.

It was during the Battle of Shrewsbury in 1403 that English surgeon John Bradmore saved the life of young Prince Henry, son and heir to King Henry IV (1367–1413). Bradmore, who was court physician to the king, practised surgery along with other members of his family. Both his brother Nicholas and his son-in-law were surgeons. Fighting under his father's command, Prince Henry, just sixteen years old, charged into battle. The high-ranking Percy family of Northumberland had revolted against the king. They assembled an army and marched south through Cheshire into Shrewsbury, where the king's forces met them. The Battle of Shrewsbury was one of the bloodiest battles in English history. During the battle, Prince Henry perhaps lifted his visor and was wounded. However it got there, a bodkin arrow hit Henry in the face and broke under the steel of his helmet. Though the arrow had entered his cheekbone, Henry stayed on fighting for over an hour. The arrow had entered the boy's face at an angle and penetrated just left of his nose, underneath his eye. Although the young warrior had received a horrific and possibly fatal wound, he refused to leave the battle. He awaited word that his father's forces had overcome. He then went with surgeons to Kenilworth Castle for treatment, a journey of over fifty miles. It's important to point out that the litter that carried the prince would have had to navigate over a long bumpy road. The prince was surely jostled about in his carriage, no doubt causing immeasurable pain to his face. Surgeons had originally tried to pull the arrow from Henry's face by twisting it. Their attempts did nothing but add to his discomfort, as the arrow could not be successfully removed. At Kenilworth, Henry was taken under the care of John Bradmore. The physician probed the wound and measured its depth. Surgical removal of arrowheads often involved propulsion, where the arrow was forced through the skin to make an exit wound, but this was not the case with John Bradmore's treatment plan. He washed the wound and filled it with an ointment consisting of honey and elderflower. He then sealed the wound and sent Henry on his way to a nearby abbey to rest. Over the four days that the prince was resting, Bradmore designed an instrument, called the Bradmore Screw, to try to remove the arrowhead. The tool consisted of a long needle with a screwed thread at one end and a sleeve with a tip the shape of an arrowhead. The needle was then pushed through the sleeve, forcing the tip of the sleeve to open. The needle was meant to grip the arrowhead from the inside. Bradmore himself describes it as such:

> First, I made small probes from the pith of an elder, well dried and well stitched in purified linen the length of the wound. These probes were infused with rose honey. And after that, I made larger and larger probes, and so I continued to always enlarge these probes until I had the width and depth of the wound as I wished it. And after the wound was as enlarged and deep enough so that, by my reckoning, the probes reached the bottom of the wound, I prepared anew some little tongs, small and hollow, and with the width of an arrow A screw ran through the middle of the tongs, whose ends were well

rounded both on the inside and outside, and even the end of the screw, which was entered into the middle, was well rounded overall in the way of a screw, so that it should grip better and more strongly.

After clearing away the pus that had gathered in the wound, Bradmore tried to grab the arrowhead using his new tool, but the arrowhead moved further up into the nasal cavity. He then went up the prince's nose and pushed the arrowhead back down. After clearing away the blood that seeped from the wound, Bradmore's screw finally latched onto the arrowhead "By moving it to and fro, little by little, with the help of God, I extracted the arrowhead".

He then rewashed the wound, and after sewing up the inside of the young man's nose, Bradmore began the next part of his treatment. The doctor squirted white wine and then ran a bandage soaked in barley, flour, and honey into the wound. He then sealed the injury and, in two days, cleaned the wound and began the process over. Over the next twenty days, he repeated the process, cleaning the wound and allowing it to heal naturally from the inside and close. Little did Bradmore know at the time, but he had just pioneered a procedure that is still practised today in modern medicine. He was rewarded greatly for his work and granted an annuity of ten marks until his death in 1412. Although Prince Henry's life had been saved, there remained a significant scar, both physically and emotionally. All portraits of Henry, who would eventually become a great king, show only the side of his face that was not disfigured by the accident. The prince was known for being a rather untamed youth, but by the time he was crowned in 1413, he had become a disciplined and serious leader. Perhaps having such a wound and facing death had helped to turn Henry into the fierce leader who would later prevail at the Battle of Agincourt.

Before his death, John Bradmore wrote a surgical treatise called *Philomena*. Along with a full account of the treatment of Prince Henry, the text is comprised of writings on anatomy, abscesses, wound, and ulcer care, as well as dislocations. Another famous case worth noting is Bradmore's treatment of William Wynecelowe, the Master of the Royal Pavilions. Wynecelowe had made an unsuccessful attempt to end his life, resulting in two deep wounds to his abdomen, one of which was rather severe. His treatment of the Master of the Royal Pavilions lasted eighty-six days, but in the end, the patient survived.

Only two years after being crowned King of England, Henry V would again show his military might at the Battle of Agincourt. A battle of the Hundred Years' War, Henry's victory at Agincourt would make England one of the most substantial military powers in the world. The Hundred Years' War was a series of battles and conflicts that lasted from 1337–1453, well over a hundred years. The English House of Plantagenet and the French House of Valois were in constant turmoil over the right to rule France. While the English had a brave, young king at their forefront, The French were not so lucky. King Charles VI (1368–1422) of France, who had a severe mental illness, was incapacitated and would not be there to lead his troops. The Battle of Agincourt is notable for its use of the English longbow. Henry's army consisted of roughly 80% Welsh and English archers. After many failed negotiations with the French, Henry V invaded. His army marched over one hundred miles from Harfleur to Calais. The English were tired, hungry, suffering from dysentery, and greatly outnumbered by the French. But Henry was still confident. During a night filled with substantial rainfall, Henry walked through his encampment giving his troops courage on the eve of the Feast of St. Crispin Day. Part of the speech, translated into modern English, follows:

> We few, we happy few, we band of brothers! The man who sheds his blood with me shall be my brother; however humble he may be. This day will elevate his status. And gentlemen in England, still lying in their beds, we think themselves accursed because they were not here. And be in awe while anyone speaks. Who fought with us on Saint Crispin's Day.

The weapon of Henry's archers, the longbow, could be propelled over two hundred and fifty meters. Although his troops were at a disadvantage and outnumbered, Henry V still claimed victory at Agincourt. The longbow shot directly into the French cavalry, causing their horses great pain and rendering them uncontrollable. The bodkin arrow of the longbow could pierce armour and chainmail, and the French were overcome with archers firing at them. And because of the heavy rains, the already ploughed field became a sea of mud. This made it very hard for the French to walk, who were predominantly in full battle armour. If they fell in the mud, they couldn't get back up. Many sank to their knees in desperation, and there are accounts of knights drowning in their own helmets from the unrelenting mud and muck. Henry also brought with him surgeon Thomas Morstede (1380–1450). Morstede had with him a group of surgeons, apprentices, and medical men. In *A Fair Book of Surgery*, a manuscript written by Morstede in 1446, he explains that:

> A good surgeon should be experienced gained from having performed surgical procedures and seeing others do them, they should also be a keen wit, to be able to give advice, and well-mannered. Alongside the desirable attributes, a surgeon should also possess certain skills and equipment. The latter included forceps, scalpels, scissors, and probes, some of which would not be unfamiliar to a modern surgeon. He should also possess various drugs, plasters, and ointments. He should also be skilled in the treatment of wounds and abscesses and how to restore damaged tissue but also in teaching others how to manage wounds.

Part of ruling a nation during the Middle Ages meant you placed yourself at risk of dying in battle, especially if yours was a country that went to war often. And for Scottish king James IV (1473–1513), that was just the case. In 1502, the Treaty of Perpetual Peace had been signed between Scotland and its usually unruly southern neighbour, England. The English king, Henry VII, even granted the marriage of his daughter, Margaret (1489–1541), to James. But in 1509, when Henry VIII took the throne, things would change between Scotland and England. In June 1513, England invaded Scotland's ally, France and James had no choice but to retaliate. With over forty thousand men, James IV and Scotland's army invaded England from the north when the English king was in France. But Henry wasn't stupid, and he left one of his best military commanders, the Earl of Surrey (1517–1547), as well as his wife, the fierce Queen Katherine of Aragon, in charge. Katherine was the daughter of warrior Queen Isabella of Castile (1451–1504), and it was in her blood not to back down. With Katherine's help, Surrey had gathered roughly twenty-five thousand men in Northern England to meet their Scottish enemies.

As some of the Scottish king's men were deserting him, the English army moved north around Ford Castle and met the Scottish army at Branxton Hill. The Scots were poorly positioned and met with some nasty blows from the English army. The English were equipped and well trained with the longbow, as well as extensive cavalry, while the Scots struggled with a French weapon they didn't understand how to use. They weren't trained well in the new long pike, and the saturated ground of the battlefield had limited their potential even more. Meanwhile, the English were battle-ready with the bill hook arrow, which was excellent in close combat and precise in chopping the long pike in half. In what would ultimately be a suicidal charge, James IV led his army to clash with the English in a complete massacre. The Scottish king fought ferociously until the bloody end. He charged into the thick of the battle with admirable courage. He finally fell, his body littered with dozens of English arrows and his throat slashed by the infamous bill hook. James had inspired an enormous amount of devotion in his men, and they followed him to their ultimate demise. Edward Hall, an English chronicler, wrote, "The battle was cruel, none spared other, and the King himself fought valiantly".

The body of the king was removed from the mass of butchered corpses that lay on the bloody battlefield. It was embalmed and presented to the English queen. She was intent on giving the head of her enemy to her husband but was talked into sending only his slashed, blood-stained field jacket instead.

Queen Katherine's lust for victory can only be attributed to her mother, but it also gives us a grave understanding of the need for dominance on the battlefield. It helps us to understand the absolute perils of war and to appreciate further all that the battle surgeons subjected themselves to. It was Erasmus who said, "War is delightful to those who have no experience of it".

In the eyes of the physician on the battlefield, I believe these words hold a great deal of truth. And it was all in the name of the crown.

Chapter Eight

Housing the Poor, the Sick and the Insane

When it comes to the medieval hospital, there remains a great misunderstanding as to what precisely a hospital was. The earliest hospitals in the Middle Ages were those of hospitality and shelters for all. The very word, hospital, is derived from the Latin word *Hospes*, meaning host or guest. But the destruction of so many religious buildings during the English Reformation has left historians to dig through the rubble both physically and metaphorically. From the eleventh century to the middle of the 1500s, there were close to 1,300 hospitals in England alone. But sadly, most of them have been left to nothing but ruin.

In the tenth, eleventh and twelfth centuries, hospitality was an obligation, a duty, and a privilege to welcome travellers. And the earliest hospitals in England were predominantly religious houses. These were places where taking care of one's soul was just as important as taking care of their body. Most of these hospitals were for the sick or ageing patient and were often referred to as almshouses and generally followed the Benedictine Rule. Almshouses provided charity to the poor and other folks who needed assistance, be it medically or spiritually.

Saint Benedict of Nursia, the patron saint of Europe, founded the Abbey of Monte Cassino in southeast Rome in or around the year 529. The only account of Benedict is found in writings by Pope Gregory. He writes of a gentle abbot who was well disciplined. The son of a Roman noble, it is believed that he left his studies at the age of twenty. He had been sent to Rome for education but was not satisfied with the things he found there. Perhaps he was unhappy with the busyness of the bustling city.

Along with one of his nurses, Benedict left Rome for the town of Enfide, which was roughly forty miles from the city. Far above the mountains, Benedict met Romanus of Subiaco (d. 550 AD), who had been living as somewhat of a hermit in a mountain cave. After trying to understand the meaning of his journey, Benedict too, lived as a hermit for several years. Benedict would mature spiritually over this time and earned the respect of those around him as a man of honour. Benedict founded twelve monasteries throughout the town of Subiaco, and in the year 530, Monte Cassino was founded. It was here that Benedict wrote *The Benedictine Rule*, the principle rule of monks living together under an abbot. These rules were established as the founding principles for monasteries going forward. Benedict stressed that there was a moral obligation to care for the sick and destitute. His hospital in Monte Cassino became a model hospital and was the stepping stone to enforcing the Benedictine rules in caring for the needy.

Settlements of these religious communities were built to house monks, priests, and even laypeople. Together they lived a life of spiritual discipline based on the Benedictine Rule. These buildings ranged in size from communities housing several hundred to houses with only a few members. No matter the size, the brothers practised the fundamentals of the Catholic Church in their dedication to the community and the sick. Aside from being houses of prayer, monasteries have been synonymous as places of charity and giving.

The framework of the early medieval hospital was often built in the shape of a cross, a result of the influence of monastic rule. Aside from the construction of the undercroft, which was used for storage in most cases, the early almshouses were constructed around the infirmary hall. The hall, a long, narrow structure connected to the chapel, was often designed under an impressive archway, with several bays along its side. The number of bays could differ according to the size of the building. Because monks understood the importance of caring for both sexes equally, the bays would usually be separated. Even in the case of an existing structure being constructed into an almshouse, the tradition of the infirmary hall with the attached chapel remained. It was important to adhere to standard hospital construction. As hospitals grew in size, a second hall may have been added on. This was the case of St. Mary's Hospital in Dover in the fourteenth century. The interior of the infirmary hall typically presented with rows of beds down the length of the corridor. The intention was such that all patients were in plain view of the hospital chapel and could hear Mass. Early hospital beds were most likely made from simple straw pallets until the late twelfth century, when wooden beds were introduced. The centre of the infirmary hall usually boasted some form of lighting, and it's possible that lighting was provided next to each bed. Again, of the utmost importance was that one had a clear view of the altar. Although patients were expected to bring their own linens if they had them, grants were given to provide them to patients if needed. Most almshouses were meagerly furnished, with only the necessities, bedding, books, tables, and basins.

The chapel of the hospital was an essential part of the building and received the best care when it came to upkeep. A lot of funds and dedication were put into designing the hospital chapel. It was usually of quality woodwork and intricate details in both stone and wood. Grand designs were the norm, as the chapels got the most attention in both construction and alterations. Those that had windows were impressive with Norman stained glass. In the mid-thirteenth century, the chapel at St. John the Baptist in Litchfield was totally rebuilt with beautiful woodwork throughout the interior. There is also evidence to support the use of bold statues in chapels along with wall paintings. Specific clerks were designated to tend to the lights and vestments and see that the rushes on the floor be kept clean.

By the ninth century, the Benedictine way was the standard form of monastic life in Western Europe. These monasteries indeed became a dominant factor when it came to caring for the sick. Founded in the year 910, the Benedictine Abbey of Cluny, in France, set the example for the centre of relief that hospitals would become. The Benedictine monks were wholly devoted to prayer and the liturgy. This was a bit unusual in that the monks did not focus on physical labour. Instead, they were consistent in achieving a state of grace with their endless prayers. The abbey housed one of the biggest libraries in Europe and, at its glory, was the most significant monastic order in the Western world. By the 1200s, it had grown in size, reaching 656 feet, and was the largest building in the world until the construction of St. Peter's Basilica. Pope Urban II called Cluny Abbey "The Light of the World".

After the Norman Conquest, most works of mercy were done in the monastery. Englishmen have always loved travel and to visit holy shrines. Many hospitals were built along the pilgrimage routes that could house thirty people or more. And all were welcome, travellers, invalids, even lepers. St James at Horning was a popular stop for those en route to Walshingham. In the year 800, a small group of Saxon monks erected a chapel dedicated to St. Benedict near the River Bure. Although the building was destroyed, it was rebuilt in 960 by a holy man name Wulfric. In 1019, King Cnut (990 CE-1035 CE) endowed the abbey with the manors of Horning. The hospital of St James at Horning was founded in 1153, and the number of monks remained relatively consistent.

In 1148, St Bartholomew's in Smithfield became the resort of sick pilgrims, and people began to flock to the hospital shrine. St Bartholomew's was founded in 1123 by Rahere (1144), a courtier of King Henry I and an Augustinian canon regular. Rahere had come down with malaria while in Italy. He had a vivid dream that a winged beast brought him to a higher place and gave him a message from God. He was to erect a great church in London for its people. Rahere promised himself and God that if he survived, he would build a grand place for the poor in London. With the blessing of the king, Rahere began construction on what was royal property. After hearing of his divine message, Henry I granted him the use of the land. After gaining a reputation of healing, victims of epilepsy, dropsy, fever, and insanity all flocked to St. Bartholomew's. Several miracles are said to have occurred here, including the curing of serious ailments and disabilities after a visit.

Early English hospitals did not have doctors or surgeons on board. Care of patients took many forms, whether they were social or spiritual. Concern was to meet the many needs of the patient, and this was not done through highly medicalised means. This care was directly for the sick and poor as the rich would have been able to have a qualified physician treat them at their home.

While many of the early English hospitals were for people travelling and on foot, some hospitals were more houses of permanent relief. St John's of Canterbury, founded in roughly 1085, had been intended for men and women who were of ill health and may have needed a more extended stay. The blind, lame, deaf, and sick found refuge here. St. John's still has a considerable amount of upstanding to this day. The Norman architecture remains reasonably well preserved despite the destruction of so many other religious buildings throughout England. The building survived the dissolution of the monasteries and is believed to be one of the oldest surviving hospitals in England.

Kepier Hospital, founded at Gilesgate in Durham, was built for the poor. It was founded by Bishop Flambard (1060–1128), who dedicated it to God and to St. Giles, the patron saint of beggars and cripples. Scottish men, under orders from their king, destroyed part of the building, but it was refounded in 1180 by Bishop Hugh le Puiset (1125–1195). The hospital housed roughly thirteen brothers and served the poor as well as travellers on route to pilgrims. While Kepier hospital was closed in 1535 by Henry VIII, much of the building remains intact today. The hospital of St. Cross in Winchester, founded in 1136 by Henry of Blois, Bishop of Winchester (1096–1171), stays standing today. Both Kepier and St. Cross are examples of almshouses in England that gave considerable charity to the sick and destitute.

As the Shrine of St Thomas of Canterbury became the goal of travellers, it was necessary to find accommodation for them. More hospitals began to pop up along the way, including Ospringe and Strood, where "poor, weak travellers from distant places were cared for until they healed or died".

Commissioned by Henry III in 1234, Ospringe Hospital in Kent was a small foundation with a master and three brothers. The keepers of Ospringe were hospitable and welcoming to the poor and the needy who came upon it in their travels. Ospringe was a perfect example of how the sick were cared for in society during that period.

The early medieval hospital was not only a guest house but was clearly becoming an infirmary. The work of charity, as shown by St. Mary's in London, included:

> If anyone in infirm health and destitute of friends should seek admission for a term until he shall recover, let him be gladly received and assigned a bed. In regard to the poor people who are received late at night, and go forth early in the morning, let the warden take care that their feet are washed, and, as far as possible, their necessities attended to.

Standards of care for hospitals varied quite a bit, but almost all shared the holistic approach of healing the body and the soul as one. Because the Galenic approach to medicine was stressed through the importance of diet, the food offered throughout the Middle Ages at hospitals was almost always healthy. It was common for patients to be given homemade ales and wine, along with fresh-baked bread. Fresh cheese and soups were also distributed to patients to keep up their strength. The general consensus that the miasma theory held true throughout medieval Europe, and so those serving at the hospital prided themselves on keeping the air clean. Floors were continuously swept, and linens were kept clean. It was indeed the belief that a positive environment would help to ease the pain patients were in. Food, a clean, warm, and comfortable experience was the achieved outcome for patients.

One of the most famous and perhaps ideal hospitals was the hospital of St. John's in Jerusalem. The religious order that ran the hospital was often referred to as *The Hospitallers*. The Hospitallers developed in the twelfth century as a group associated with Amalfitan, an Italian hospital, in the Christian district of Jerusalem. After the conquest of Jerusalem in 1099, the Hospitallers became a military and religious order that was charged with defending the Holy Land. St John's in Jerusalem was entirely staffed by medical practitioners, both doctors and surgeons, bloodletters and brethren. The medical practitioners made the same morning and evening rounds that physicians make today in a hospital setting. All who worked at the hospital were required to live by a strict code of obedience and chastity.

The brethren prided themselves on treating their patients as Christ would have. Everything from beds to a healthy meal was given to patients in addition to their full attention. An anonymous visitor to the hospital wrote of the piety and commitment of the brothers:

> It has happened on a number of occasions that when the space proves insufficient for the multitude of the suffering, the dormitory of the brethren is taken over by the sick, and the brethren themselves sleep on the floor.

Like so many medieval hospitals in England, the sacrament was given as the first step in restoring one's health. In 1215, an ordinance was passed that one must confess before being admitted to a hospital, as cleansing the soul was the first step towards healing. But the Hospitallers believed that everyone should be accepted, and no one was turned away. Muslims or Jews who came to them in a time of need were warmly taken in. The same anonymous visitor wrote this on his observation of such attentiveness:

> The sick are gathered together in this house out of every nation, every social condition, and both sexes so that by the mercy of the Lord the number of lords increase in proportion to the multitude of languages. Indeed, knowing well that …

And it is here that the visitor makes a biblical reference "The Lord invites all to salvation and wishes none to perish (Ezek 18:32), men of pagan religion find mercy within this holy house if they flock thither, and even Jews".

Wounded soldiers were also brought to the hospital to be tended to. While not all hospitals would provide this sort of care, along with a warm, clean bed and food, St. John's of Jerusalem certainly seemed to be the model medieval hospital.

As with most medicine, it seems that England was a bit behind the times when it came to the hospital. At least when compared to those in Italy. Santa Maria of Nuova in Florence, founded in 1288, is one of the most critical institutions in Italy and remains functioning today. At the time of its building, the hospital boasted both a female and male ward and was said to be able to accommodate up to two hundred patients. They also had an impressive medical staff on board, including doctors, surgeons, and an eye doctor. Most of the hospitals in Florence were extraordinary, as they served fresh food and drink and were known for their cleanliness and learned staff. The larger Italian communities of not only Florence but Padua and Venice genuinely organised the city hospital. These institutions enabled the smooth running of the business from all aspects. They protected those from all social classes, including orphans, the sick, and the poor. What made them so different from the monastic hospitals was they had university-educated physicians as a part of their staff. Another of these was Ca Granda Ospedale Maggiore Policlinico in Milan, founded by Duke Francesco Sforza in 1456. The hospital still fully functions today and remains one of the oldest hospitals in Italy. The Hotel-Dieu in Paris is perhaps one of the oldest hospitals in the city. Founded by Saint Landry (d 661) in 625 CE, it cared for many of the city's poor who came for aid. Like most hospitals of the time, the link between loyalty and medical care was secure. Hotel-Dieu was truly an institution for the poor and sick.

The chief building period for hospitals was over by the late 1300s. By the early 1400s, the assistance of women in childbirth was soon to be recognised as a vital hospital charity. The deed of the Holy Trinity in Salisbury said, "lying in women are cared for until they are delivered, recovered and churched".

In London, St Mary's and St. Bartholomew's instructed that if the mother died in childbirth, the child would be cared for until age seven. The earliest homes for women included St. Katherine's in London, where the sisters would provide for fatherless children and widows. Orphans in danger or deserted children could be adopted into the hospital family. St Leonard's in York ministered to quite a few orphans where education was provided, as well as grammar and music.

The construction of hospitals began to change starting around the year 1350. They were enlarged, and often separate rooms were added for patrons having a temporary stay, where they awaited a visit from the warden. Preparations were also made to house long term patients, those that were lame or blind or had perhaps lost a limb and needed constant care. Separate buildings were provided for the working brethren as well as those who may be retiring from monastic life. Overall, the initial infirmary hall type construction was slowly declining. Economic fluctuations, as well as spiritual decline throughout England, caused changes in building structure. Many of the earlier built hospitals had begun to deteriorate as there was a lack of revenue, and the resources on hand had started to deplete. Fires were often a cause of destruction as well as the chaos of foreign raids.

By the fifteenth century, church revenue had begun to decline seriously, and there was not much funding left for any repairs to the buildings. St. Giles and St. Thomas the Martyr in Canterbury had stretched their budget terribly, leaving almost nothing. This was often the case as things were mismanaged, and too much money was poured into additions and repairs that left the Church budget dry. In 1375, some hospitals had reduced themselves to such poverty that they could hardly support themselves any longer. In the case of St Mary's in Chichester, a commission to look into and repair church defects was drawn up in 1382. However, this was only around one hundred years after the initial construction of the building, and there had been no recorded evidence that anything needed repair. Churches began to see less and less donations from the public, and royal support, as well, was starting to weaken. The monarch had also begun to propose long lists of folks who were granted lifelong allowances of food and shelter. These impositions cost the religious institutions a great deal as some of these allowances were careless and irresponsible. These long-term residents who didn't need the hospital as a necessity had begun to take up beds that were needed for the sick. Poor administration by monastic overseers had started to affect the hospitals as well. Wasteful spending and the use of goods were caused by the increasing dishonesty of the abbey masters. This led to a reduction in the quality of products and services essential for both staff and the patients. The wardens began to take more than their share of things and this, in turn, left less for the brethren. In 1328, at God's House, in Southampton, there was a particular issue about the quality of their baked bread. There always seemed to be enough high-quality bread for the warden's visit but not for others. When the warden, Gilbert de Wyggeton would visit, his meals were much more desirable than those served to the staff. It was also noted that much more wine was purchased during his visits, along with fresh meats and fruits. This put tremendous strain on the finances of the hospital.

It was also noted that wardens and masters enjoyed the resources of the hospitals for their own personal use. In 1359, St Bartholomew's in Gloucester was all but pillaged by the masters. Corn, silver, jewels, and household utensils were said to have been dissipated. Extravagant clothing and furniture had also provided extreme pleasure for the master. In fact, by the time of the Reformation, most hospitals had the addition of a separate house for their master. These quarters were usually private, and any obligation of the masters to share sleeping quarters with the brothers was being overlooked. Master's houses were often given elaborate fabrics and non-essential alterations. Some of their quarters were also partitioned into separate rooms, including personal kitchens.

Over time, these added comforts for the master of the hospital became the object of envy to the brethren and sisters. These same things were expected and soon given to the staff. Certain priests began to receive special privileges, including their own suitable living quarters next to the Church. These residences were often elaborate in nature, including plastered walls and grand fireplaces. Hospitals began building private chambers for nobles and upper-class guests as they looked for higher standards than simple folk. This increase in privacy also called for a change in the infirmary hall itself. Partitions were constructed to provide more disclosed areas for patients. St. Nicholas in Salisbury began to make changes in the fifteenth century as the south side of the building was made into a separate patient area, and further rooms were built. The north porch of the structure was also turned into different quarters.

Criticism had begun to pour in regarding the lax behaviour of the monasteries. At St John the Baptist in Northampton, there were reports of extravagant food and clothing being used and that the brethren were having "drinking parties" in their chambers. This criticism only added to the problems of low resources and spiritual decline.

The mid-fourteenth century brought about an important turning point in the construction of the medieval hospital. The infirmary hall was being built in a manner that divided its patients, and not everyone was housed under one roof, as they had been previously. Founders of the newer almshouses ensured that they were not neglected, so specific ordinances were drawn up to guard against any threats or mismanagement. As merchants and tradesmen became more involved with the construction of the hospitals, there was more concern in protecting their investments. The newer buildings were generally smaller but also adequately endowed, and money was set aside for any upcoming repairs. Annual reports were drawn up on the details of the property as well. The construction of the newer hospitals followed the general outline of a group of buildings surrounding a courtyard. Church officials who were in service to the crown began to accumulate money, and a way of showing off their riches was to build new hospitals. Attention to detail was apparent with lavish construction and luxuriously carved boards in the gables. Privacy was still an essential factor in the more modern hospitals, as private quarters with fireplaces were built. The standard of personal living was increased as well as familiar comfort. A garderobe was built into each individual dwelling, and heating was improved with larger fireplaces.

It wasn't until the construction of Savoy Hospital, as part of Savoy Palace, that the medieval English hospital began to catch up with its European neighbours. Henry VII had left endowments and instructions for it to be built in his will. In or after the year 1512, his son King Henry VIII gave the go-ahead for the building to begin. Savoy Hospital would be grand in its structure and the first in England to have a permanent medical staff. With rooms assembled in the shape of a cross, the hospital boasted a chapel and separate lodgings for staff. The king wanted to provide 100 beds for patients with a view of the altar as the first traditional hospitals had been built. The Savoy was constructed for the specific purpose of temporary relief. Patrons were given one night's food and lodging unless they were sick enough to be admitted on a more prolonged basis. Upon admittance to the Savoy, a patient was given a hot bath and their clothes and belongings cleaned. Separate roles were appointed to all staff, and a matron, along with twelve other women, were added. The hospital also had an impressive garden as hospitals for the poor relied heavily on herbalists. These herbalists were often women who were typically older with a lot of domestic experience. The hospital developed a delousing program, had water piped in, and an operative waste disposal system was built. English physicians believed that worms of various shapes originated in the gut when the organs contained an excess of phlegmatic humours. Worms, and probably lice, were treated using pungent plants such as wormwood, which would not only kill the parasites but give the patient a nasty case of diarrhoea. Patients may have also been subjected to treatment with mercury or could have been deloused using a simple nit comb.

Aside from the almshouse that cared for the sick and travelling of England, there was another type of hospital that catered to an entirely different cause; leprosy. I think it's important to touch briefly on the mass hysteria that can arise when the word leprosy is mentioned. Modern-day shows us a very different picture of the disease. In truth, what medical professionals have learned about the disease should put us at great ease. We have always been told of the horrors of leprosy and the leper hospital. We have been convinced that total seclusion was the best treatment for the affliction, but this simply wasn't the case. As you will see, the actual leper hospitals were very unlike the romantic notion that history has given them.

Leprosy was documented to be most active between the eleventh century through to the mid to end of the thirteenth century. The popularity of leper hospitals spread over those 200 years, and although it's hard to pinpoint precisely, historians believe there were around 300 leper houses in England at the time. Although most lived in hospitals, it wasn't uncommon for lepers to live in the community as well. These hospitals were cautious about who they accepted, and it wasn't heard of to have an admittance fee charged. Patients were also expected to adhere to the strict rules of the Benedictine monks, or they could be asked to leave. Hospitals catered to the urban areas, especially the areas surrounding the city. Leprosy seemed to affect the more built-up communities, and so hospitals were generally funded by the royal family or important members of the clergy. Leper hospitals were usually built on the major routes that led into the cities and appeared as a refreshing beacon of light at the gates of the cities.

The first leper hospital was founded by Matilda of Scotland (1080–1118), the queen of English king Henry I. Known as *Good Queen Matilda*, she was a deeply pious and caring woman. She was the epitome of holiness and had a keen interest in serving the poor and those with leprosy. She founded the hospital of St. Giles in Holborn and could be found washing the feet of the lepers and kissing their hands. Her acts angered some, including her brother, who was revolted by what she was doing. Matilda claimed that in kissing the lepers, she was kissing the skin of Christ, and it mattered not to her that they were diseased. Her outlook is a testament to how many saw the connection of Christ to the leper. Several other prominent leper hospitals began to pop up around the edges of London, including Les Lokes in Southwark, constructed in 1227. Lepers in most of the hospitals were overseen by a civic warden, who managed the home. The House of Hackney was built around 1330, and hospitals in Knightsbridge and Mile End were both constructed around 1475.

The general thought process surrounding leprosy has significantly been misrepresented. History has loved to dramatize it, claiming it is a disease in which the victims should be utterly secluded from everyday life. Due in part to the Reformation so much was lost as far as text or medical documentation regarding day-to-day life in the leper hospitals. And during the beginning of the twentieth century, leprosy was assumed to be very contagious, so physicians looked to the Middle Ages for a better understanding. So much information was distorted that a construed view of leper victims emerged. They were seen as social outcasts that terrified the public and should be kept with outlaws. These embellishments are due mostly in part to the imagination of several artists and historical writers during the 1920s. One of the artists who should be credited for his beautiful watercolour paintings is Richard Cooper (1885–1957). He painted in and around the year 1912, and his painting, *People Scrambling to Get Away from a Leper*, depicts this very thing; people of an unnamed medieval town scrambling furiously to retreat from the leper who is wandering through the streets. But like so much else concerning the romanticism surrounding the disease in the early 1900s, Cooper's breathtaking painting is a great exaggeration.

History depicts several images with Christ healing the leper, and it is clearly stated in the Bible that this was the case. In Mark 1:40–45, Jesus heals the leper and sends him back out into society. But instead of obeying Jesus and keeping quiet, the leper tells all who will listen, causing a flood of people to flock to him to hear of this miracle. However, it was seen as a distraction, and Jesus retreated. He took the place of the outcast, substantially changing positions with the leper. Several biblical picture books show Christ as the leper himself. Christ was not afraid to lay his hands upon a leper, and there is an excellent connection to lepers being viewed as Christ-like or very close to Christ. Leprosy was seen as a purgatorial suffering here on earth. Physicians were regularly encouraged to reassure their patients diagnosed with leprosy that they would go straight to heaven and didn't have to worry about going through purgatory.

Leper hospitals were reported to be well-stocked with goods to care for their patients. Inhabitants of the hospital were given healthy food as nourishment as well as clean linens. Patients were also instructed to pray for their caregivers and the community regularly. This encouraged monetary donations as it was expected of the public to care for the lepers in their community. And by giving your funds to an institution, it was a guarantee that several of those, close to Christ, would be praying for you. Leper patients were also encouraged to be self-sufficient. Patients were given light duties, such as gardening or tending to livestock around the hospital. And they were given the "prescription" of daily exercise.

The predisposed notion that we have today of the leper being shunned from society and forced to live alone can be attributed to a bible passage in Leviticus. The passage mentions that infected people should first be examined by a priest and then sent to live away until fully healed. But in reality, leprosy is only mildly contagious, and you need to be in close contact with the victim to risk infection. You need to be close enough to breathe in mucus or saliva water droplets. It's also necessary to understand that the term leprosy was used as a rather broad brush for people with simple skin diseases. It wasn't suggested that you should actually leave town until your symptoms became quite visible. It could often take years for the disease to progress. So people could have been plagued with a case of psoriasis or another skin condition, which certainly would have looked like leprosy if left untreated. But simply because those diagnosed were asked to live apart did not mean they were shunned entirely from public life. Lepers were allowed to enter towns to ask for food or beg for alms, and they were indeed allowed to go on pilgrimage to pray for healing. It is only apparent today, by looking at the skeletal remains of lepers, what the disease would do in the last stages. Human skeletons show the results of nerve damage in missing appendages or damage to the nasal cavity.

There are several depictions of the leper ringing his bell as he wanders through town. As I explained in a previous chapter, the bell was more of a way of announcing oneself because he or she most likely lost their voice in the advancing stages of the disease. The reluctance of English doctors to accept any medical text that was new or suggested a different thought process would hold them back centuries when it came to accurately diagnosing leprosy. Because documents from Muslim countries were all but ignored, it may help us to understand why there was such a large number of lepers in medieval England. The scholar Avicenna spoke in detail about leprosy in his medical text, *The Canon of Medicine*. But it wasn't until almost two hundred years after he wrote it that anyone paid much attention to it. So perhaps those with leprosy weren't afflicted after all and were just suffering from another skin condition. But by using archaic analysis, English doctors most likely gave a lot of false diagnoses.

It's relatively easy to understand how people thought leprosy was more contagious than it actually was. Because medieval medicine focused primarily on the miasma theory for an explanation as to why infectious diseases spread, it made perfect sense in the case of leprosy. It is known today why the mouth and nose were affected by the disease. We can understand how the condition ate away at the flesh in and around the oral cavity. Medieval doctors certainly knew that leprosy affected the mouth but just didn't understand precisely how. The effects of leprosy caused bone erosion and dental loss. Periodontal disease was very prevalent among leper victims as there was considerable wasting away of the tooth structure and soft tissue. And it is understood today that periodontal disease is one of the leading causes of halitosis. Halitosis is mentioned as one of the key symptoms in people suffering from leprosy in the Middle Ages. So, if we consider that the bad air theory convinced people, it only makes sense to think that one's foul breath would be a significant factor in this case. And while lepers were generally tolerated when allowed to enter public areas, it didn't mean that there weren't cries of protest either.

During the reign of the English king Edward III, there was much public protest about letting lepers wander freely. The king did issue a royal proclamation that the foul breath of the leper was indeed a threat to others. He declared that anyone who was diagnosed with leprosy was to leave the city within fifteen days "and betake themselves to places in the country, solitary, and notably distant from the city and suburbs".

Other documents record the eviction of lepers, including one in 1273. A 1327 municipal document states that a leper named John Mayn was given reported warnings to leave town and not return, or he would be enclosed in a pillory. However, the law generally left lepers alone if they did not interfere with the public and stayed towards the edges of roadways, or better yet, only came out at night. Nonetheless, in keeping pace with the intent of the leper hospitals, there was believed to have been a feeling of generosity and support among the people of England. There was some sense of an obligation to take care of the sick and diseased because the spiritual benefits were aplenty, and of course, this was the Christ-like thing to do.

Treatment of the mad or insane during the Middle Ages remained a bit of a conundrum because mental illness was probably one of the things that physicians understood the least. If your sanity was at risk, more emphasis was put on how to deal with your lands rather than your illness. This was especially true if you were of noble birth. Treatment and dealings differed. If you were on the lower rung of society, you could expect little to no treatment for your illness. The belief in demonic possession was so prevalent during the Middle Ages that most psychiatric conditions were blamed on it. You could have been viewed as spiritually bankrupt as well as mad. Whether your treatment was of medical or divine intervention, the outcome was to get you to recover and return to your senses.

Mental illness had been recognised as far back as the Ancient Greeks, and it was certainly mentioned in the Bible. It was possible that going mad was viewed as a curse from God, or in the case of the Greeks, a curse from the gods on humans who had displeased them. Hippocrates and Galen did try to name some of the conditions that they deemed unfit. Epilepsy, mania, melancholy and humoral imbalance were several reasons why you might be afflicted. In the case of hysteria, Hippocrates decided that this was usually a woman's problem as they were upset more easily over trivial things. The wandering womb was a belief that the uterus had become displaced and that it was the common cause of hysteria in women. Although it was a condition that came from ancient Greek theology, it was a popular theory through the 1600s. Aretaues, a philosopher from the second century, wrote that the uterus could move from its rightful place and float about through the body. The uterus was believed to be a living thing inside the woman that could move about like an animal, causing symptoms of hysteria.

A law was enacted in the thirteenth century in which a "natural born idiot", one who had been deemed insane since birth, was protected by law. The care of the insane was usually left to the family, but if they were unable to care for you, a provision was made by the crown. A legally insane person's best interest was at hand, and it was the primary care of the realm, and the community, to see that you were well taken care of. The problem was, of course, that there was little to any understanding about mental health in the Middle Ages. There were very few hospitals that made it a point to care for the insane as the crown was more concerned with your lands. Part of the law in caring for someone with mental illness meant that your estate was protected under the kingdom.

During the reign of Edward I of England (1239–1307), under *Praerogativa Regis* (The Royal Prerogative), a distinction was made between a natural-born idiot and a lunatic. A natural-born idiot was incompetent from birth, but a lunatic was declared insane at some point in their lives. If you had always been mad, your lands would be held in wardship by the crown. They would remain so until you died, and your estates would be passed on to an heir. In the case of the lunatic, the realm still provided for you and your family but did so without taking your lands. The rational thought behind this was that you had acquired your properties during a period of sanity, and so you should be able to keep them until you had your wit about you again. For the king to decide your case, you were taken before a jury of about twelve men and questioned. Was the person insane? If so, when did it start, and were there any periods of lucidity? Did the person own any lands, and if so, who was their heir? The alleged insane were given a chance to speak for themselves and to answer any questions. These questions were typically put gently, and the person was given a series of quick memory tests combined with an assessment of necessary skills. Once the mental capacity of a patient had been established, settlements were decided, and lands distributed accordingly. The council was more apt to name a natural fool because, of course, that meant more money for the crown, and in roughly 80% of cases, one was deemed a "natural idiot". The insane were usually given food, clothing, shoes, and a bed that would be charged to their estate. The care of the insane was rooted in who would care for your lands rather than what to do with you. In the case of most married women, they weren't typically given an inquisition as it was assumed that a women's husband would deal with her mental state.

You were of little importance to the crown if you didn't own lands and were most often left to your own devices. This was frequently the case with the poor, who were left to wander and beg. Most peasants were considered to be simple-minded people, and because your social rank declared your position, it was assumed that those with nobility required more thought to do their job. Because most peasants had little access to a physician, they turned to prayer for healing. If you were considered useful enough to be treated by a doctor, your treatments would include diet, exercise, possibly being bled, and most importantly, not doing anything that would cause you to get passionate.

If a member of the monarchy went mad, the kingdom went to great lengths to ensure that they were treated with the best care to assure a speedy recovery. Such was the case with Charles VI of France, Henry VI of England, and Juana of Castile (1479–1555).

Charles VI was crowned King of France at the age of eleven. He came to power when France was desperate for a strong leader after political unrest in the country. France was also years deep into the Hundred Years' War with England. He was given a proper education and suffered no signs of illness during his childhood, but France's hope that their new king would be a saviour proved wrong. At the age of 23, in April 1392, the king's illness began with a mysterious fever that caused him to start to lose his hair. He suffered occasional bouts of fever from then on and began to behave in a confused manner. It was in August of that same year that King Charles seemed to have lost his mind during a military expedition. Travelling with his men, he was startled by the loud clanking of one of his pages dropping a lance. The king withdrew his sword in defence. He began to swing his blade wildly through the air and proceeded to kill four of his knights in cold blood. He was eventually restrained by his men and brought to Paris on an ox cart as he lay speechless. His court physician,

Guillaume de Harcigny (1300–1393), at ninety-two years old, played an important role in attempting to help the king recover. But the king had fallen into a complete stupor. While it is reported that he wept greatly when he understood he had killed his own men, his mental health was clearly at stake. Attempts by his surgeons were made to cure him as they drilled holes in his skull, hoping to relieve some pressure. Whether or not this helped is unknown, but we know he suffered a relapse in 1395. He no longer recognised his queen and had forgotten his own name. His attacks of insanity happened regularly, and though he had small intervals of rationality, the uncertainty of his temper was alarming. From 1395 to 1396, the king began to make claims that he was St. George himself. He was seen running about his living quarters, darting in and out of rooms until he would collapse in utter exhaustion. He closed himself in his chambers, threatening to attack anyone who tried to help him. He urinated on himself and would damage his belongings in his fits. The king was also found on several occasions to be running through his gardens completely naked. In 1405, he spent several months refusing to bathe and threatening to kill anyone who touched him, even after contacting lice. Charles convinced himself that he was made of glass and demanded that he have iron rods sewn into his clothing so he would not shatter. His physicians resorted to trying to scare him by ordering some of his men to paint their faces and attempt to startle the king. It was this illness and the absence of a strong king which would significantly contribute to France's defeat at the Battle of Agincourt. Modern attempts to diagnose the mysterious disease of the French King have claimed it may have been encephalitis. It certainly would have made sense in explaining his bizarre behaviour. Encephalitis is known to cause a change in personality. Some medical authorities have suggested that the king may have suffered from a disease called porphyria. Porphyria, though rare, is a hereditary disease that had been diagnosed in some of Charles's ancestors. It is believed to be painful, resulting in an inflammation of the bowels and weakness in the limbs. The king's mother, Joan of Bourbon (1338–1377), was said to be unstable in mind and suffered a nervous breakdown after the birth of her seventh child. Louis of Guyenne (1397–1415), eldest son of Charles, also had questionable mental capabilities. Louis died for reasons unknown, and his brother Charles VII (1403–1461) became the successor to the throne. He, too, had odd phobias and noted psychotic episodes.

It is entirely possible that some sort of mental instability may have been passed down further by Catherine of Valois (1401–1437), daughter of the king. For when she married Henry V and gave birth to the future King of England, he too would suffer mental illness.

Henry VI succeeded to the crown of England when he was less than a year old. He too, inherited the Hundred Years' War along with setbacks in France and squabbling between nobles in his kingdom. Known for being a melancholy young man who behaved rather childishly, Henry suffered his first recorded mental breakdown in the summer of 1453. With what started with a fever, Henry went into a fit while at a hunting lodge in Wiltshire. He went into a state of withdrawal and was found to be physically and mentally catatonic. He found himself no longer able to walk or talk and couldn't even hold his head up. He was described as being slumped over like a rag doll. He seemed indifferent to what went on around him. Three months into his insanity, after several long years of waiting, the queen gave birth to a healthy baby boy. The baby was presented to the king in hopes of recognition and a blessing. But the king hadn't any idea who the child was and could not be stirred from his stupor. He no longer recognised his queen and was being spoon-fed by his attendants. Royal physicians tried a regiment of medications, baths, and enemas along with being bled, but the king didn't stir. His head was shaved in desperation to rid the brain of the black bile that physicians were sure was causing his upset. These symptoms were almost identical to what happened to his grandfather, King Charles of France. Henry was attended to, day and night, and was spared illness and given a proper diet by his men. It wasn't until December 1454 that the king began to show signs of recovery. He recognised the queen at this point, and when his child was brought to him, he was overjoyed. The monarch appeared to have suffered another attack in the fall of 1455, where he again became detached from reality. He also lost interest in the politics of his kingdom.

During the War of the Roses, Henry would continue to suffer from attacks of mental illness. In July 1460, King Henry VI was captured and then released by Yorkists at the Second Battle of St. Albans. But it was clear that the king was suffering yet another bout of insanity as he was laughing and singing merrily while the battle raged on. Ousted from his throne in February 1461, Henry and his queen fled to Scotland. After wandering as a fugitive in the forests, he was eventually seated back on the throne when Edward IV was in exile. But his second reign was short-lived, and he was taken prisoner at the Tower of London once Edward returned to reclaim his throne. In May 1471, Henry VI was found dead in the tower, believed to have been murdered.

Juana of Castile, sister of Katherine of Aragon, was sometimes referred to as The Mad Queen. Throughout her early teens, she wasn't the picture of piety her mother had hoped for. She even refused communion on several occasions, an unthinkable gesture. Juana, a youthful and smart young lady, was married at the age of sixteen to Philip I of Flanders (1478–1506). Philip was known for his incredibly good looks, which no doubt was a plus for Juana. Despite being a beauty herself, Juana could not keep her husband faithful to the marriage bed, which infuriated her. When Philip left to return for Flanders, Juana was pregnant and in a complete state of misery. She began to fall apart mentally and cried herself to sleep at night. She began to refuse food and was said to throw herself into walls. Juana's mother, Queen Isabella, forbade Juana from following her husband to Flanders. Confined to her rooms, Juana began to pace back and forth all hours of the day, making no sense when she spoke, and still, she refused to eat. Together Juana and Philip had six children. She began showing signs of being unwell as early as 1504 when her mother was ill, and in November of that year, she officially became Queen Regent of Castile when her mother passed. The pivot point in Juana's life was when her beloved husband died. Though he could not stay faithful to her, Juana was head over heels in love with him. Philip was only twenty-eight when he died of typhoid fever, although in her paranoia, Juana believed he had been poisoned. Juana was devastated and let her kingdom fall to ruins. It was her son Charles that took over the monarchy from his distraught mother. In her grief and mental instability, Juana stayed by her dead husband's body for an alarming amount of time. The widow Juana still had problems accepting her husband's death even after he had prepared for burial. She ordered her husband's casket to be opened and began an unhealthy habit of hugging and kissing him. She also made it clear that she was to be accompanied by Philip's coffin wherever she went. And her jealousy over the other women in his life plagued her even after his death. She was careful not to let any other women near his casket. She went on this way for a year until she finally agreed to have him reburied outside her window. Historians have gathered that Juana suffered from a depressive disorder, psychosis, or a case of schizophrenia. She died in her seventies of natural causes and was buried next to her beloved.

While peasants could not afford proper treatment by a physician in the event of mental illness, they were at least given the hope of divine intervention. After his death, Henry VI was revered as a saint to whom many would pray for a cure to insanity. Many miracles were attributed to the king, and he became informally regarded as a martyr. The present King of England, Henry VII, had begun compiling a list of the miracles attributed to him so he could start the canonization process for his predecessor. Several holy acts had been accredited to Henry VI, including the curing of a young girl who suffered from cervical lymphadenitis. The girl was said to have been healed by a laying on of hands by the king. Henry also interceded in the execution of a man who was being unjustly hung. With the king's hands between the rope and the accused man's throat, it is said that he kept the man alive, for he was revived after being left for dead. It was in a time when peasants sought out divine intervention and miracles, and relics such as the king's offered great hope. Demonic possession was still a very real and frightening event, especially to people with little to no education. The idea of intervention through God was often their only means of survival.

St. Dymphna of Geel, a seventh century saint from Ireland, is a source of great comfort still today. Dymphna's story involves tales of incest and murder at the hands of her father. She was said to be a bright and beautiful child who chose a vow of chastity upon entering her adolescence. She had pledged herself to a life with Christ. However, after the death of her beloved mother, things began to fall apart for her. After her father failed to find a new wife, his thoughts turned to his own daughter. On advice from her priest, she fled. Finding refuge in Geel, what is today modern Belgium, Dymphna established a home for those suffering from mental illness. Sadly, her father, who was irate at his daughter's behaviour, tracked her down. Upon finding her, he murdered her priest and severed his daughter's head. She was fifteen years old. She was profoundly mourned and praised for her good works and was canonised in 1247. A church was built in her honour during the mid-fourteenth century in Geel.

Disturbed individuals began to flock to the site and claim great miracles. The community of Geel, showing great compassion for the peasants, constructed a building to house them. Soon the residents of

Geel welcomed the mentally ill into their own homes while they visited the shrine of St. Dymphna. This tradition would continue for roughly 500 years. On 15 May, what was known as St. Dymphna's Feast Day, her relics were carried out to show the public. The insane, as well as those that cared for them, would flock to the relics and pray for healing. St. Dymphna is known as the patron saint of the mentally ill and those surviving sexual assault.

Nearly every country in Europe had such shrines that the insane would visit in hopes of a cure. There are records of them in Ireland, Scotland, England, and Germany. In France, the shrines of St. Menou, or Menulphe, and St. Dizier were visited from early times by the insane. The shrine of St. Menou at Mailly-sur-Rose was exceptionally well known, and a house was erected there to care for the mentally unstable. St. Dizier, which was believed to have been named after Desiderius of Fontenelle, ran a state of affairs much like those in Geel. Members of the community came together to embrace and care for the feeble-minded. There was an asylum for people who had a mental disease in Metz, France, in 1100 and one at Elbing near Danzig in 1320.

Respected church leaders may not have been nobles, but they were thought highly of. If they fell ill, all attempts were made to help them. In 1292, Thomas de Capella, rector at Bletchingdon, had reportedly gone mad. The Bishop of Lincoln, Oliver Sutton, saw to it that he was well taken care of. A guardian was appointed to him, and when the rector went missing, a party was sent out immediately to find him. The Bishop appointed him a coadjutor or assistant who would help to care for him and help him with his responsibilities.

Though there weren't many, England did have a small number of hospitals dedicated to helping the mentally ill. In 1247, the Priory of St. Mary of Bethlehem was founded. It became known as Bethlehem Hospital and was initially devoted to healing sick paupers. The hospital, built in the city of London, was constructed as a single storey building, covering about two acres. It was centred around a courtyard chapel. There were twelve cell-like areas for the patients, along with a kitchen and exercise yard. The monks of St Mary's had begun to understand that there were patients who required a different kind of care. They recognised the symptoms of mental illness as a separate disease. In 1346, the city of London agreed to take over things at the hospital when it began to struggle. Patients included people with not only mental illness but learning disabilities, epilepsy, and dementia. The hospital was a place to go for those who were poor and believed to be dangerous. Often, they lacked friends or family who were willing to support them. Bethlehem hospital had a mixture of ways they saw fit to help someone.

Religious devotion was more critical, along with different forms of corporal punishment believed to be beneficial. Isolation was also thought to help one find their wits once again. Inventory reports speak of manacles, chains, and locks, as well as stocks. However, it is not clear if these devices were actually used to restrain patients. In the fourteenth century, the hospital got the nickname *Bedlam* which was a word used to describe madness, chaos, and irrational nature. Sir William Dugdale (1605–1686) writes in his book *Monasticon Anglicanum* of an English asylum known as Barking Church Hospital built near the Tower of London in 1371. Robert Denton, a chaplain, had obtained a license from Edward III to found a hospital in the parish of Barking Church. It was to be for "poor priests and the men and women in the sad city who suddenly fall into a frenzy and lose their memory, who was to reside there until cured; with an oratory to the said hospital to the invocation of the Blessed Virgin Mary".

There are many records of institutions for the insane throughout Europe. However, Spain was really the first country to organize specialised institutions for the mentally ill and perhaps did so more than any other country. The origins of the first hospital established for the insane dates back to 1409 in Valencia. Joan-Gilabert Jofre (1350–1417), a Mercedarian priest, was on his way to give a Lenten sermon in February 1409 when he encountered a group of unruly children hitting and making fun of an insane man. Father Jofre broke up the assault and took the man to a nearby convent to recover. The incident inspired him to speak of the treatment of the insane in his sermon the following day:

> In this city, there are many and very important pious and charitable initiatives. However, one very necessary one is lacking, that is, a hospital or house where the innocent and frenzied would be drawn together because many poor, innocent and frenzied people wander through this city. They suffer great hardships of hunger and cold and harm, because due to their innocence and rage, they do not know how

to earn their living nor ask for the maintenance they need for their living. Therefore, they sleep in the streets and die from hunger and cold and many evil person, who do not have God in their conscience hurt them and point to where they are sleeping, they injure and kill and abuse some innocent women. It also occurs that the frenzied poor hurt many of the persons who are out wandering through the city. These things are known in the entire city of Valencia. Thus, it would be a very holy thing and work for Valencia to build a hostel or hospital where such insane or innocent persons would be housed so that they would not be wandering through the city and could not hurt nor be hurt.

Jofre's sermon moved so many of his parishioners that merchants and craftsmen provided the funds and the labour to build the hospital. In 1410, Antipope Benedict XIII (1328–1423) authorised the building as a place to care for the innocent souls, calling it *Hospital de los Inocentes* (Hospital of the Innocents). The hospital in Valencia was a complete success, and its birth began a movement that spread throughout Spain. Asylums were founded in Saragossa in 1425, in Seville in 1435, and Valladolid in 1436. They were also established in Toledo by the end of the century. The Pazzerella at Rome was founded during the sixteenth century by Ferrantez Ruiz and the Bruni, father and son, all three Navarrese. In its compassion, this hospital for the insane received patrons of whatever nation they were from.

The dissolution of the monasteries in England was by far one of the most radical events in the country's history. Because monastic houses had acquired tremendous wealth throughout the eleventh and twelfth centuries in the form of both land estates and tithes, by the sixteenth century, they owned almost a quarter of the nation's land. Throughout Europe, growing dissatisfaction with the position of religious life was evident. Criticism of monastic wealth was spreading and duly noted in the writings of Erasmus. Although he was a Catholic, Erasmus raised some critical questions when it came to the way of life in the monasteries. What had once been places of great charity had now become greedy. He felt that they profited too much by using the worship of relics and the dependence of religious pilgrimages to support their cause. The 1529 Act of Parliament under the reign of Henry VIII passed reform against the said abuses in the Catholic Church. Many felt the religious monasteries and almshouses had ceased to play a role in the spiritual existence of the country. It was observed that the strict observance of Benedictine rule had become weak and lacklustre. As more and more monasteries began to fall into debt, the standard of piety was waning. Laws of obligations regarding not only housing but communal eating had not been strictly enforced for quite some time.

The king, along with his chief advisor, Thomas Cromwell, saw this as a way to move forward in their press for reformation and to benefit the crown financially. They regarded the wealth of the monasteries to be excessive and obscene, and soon they became the target of the king's hostility. With the Protestant movement sweeping throughout much of Europe, Henry declared himself head of the new Church of England. His growing displeasure with the Catholic Pope came to a head when he was refused a declaration of nullity regarding his first marriage to Katherine of Aragon. The king married his second wife, Anne Boleyn, in addition to creating his new role as head of the Church of England. The monasteries and hospitals throughout the country now had to swear their allegiance to the king. He was the new royal authority, and if there was any opposition, it was seen as an act of treason. Friars were imprisoned, some in unfavourable conditions, and others executed for high treason.

Cromwell, under the authority of the king, began an inventory of the endowments of the monasteries. The reports that found their way back to him were mostly negative, with claims of explicit doings. There were reports of monks accepting cash for birth girdles and other religious articles. The behaviour and wealth of the religious leaders were of great offence to Cromwell. In 1535, the *Suppression of Religious Houses Act* was passed. All property and income from the offending monasteries would be dissolved and turned over to the Crown. Roofs, gutters, and plumbing were torn down as a way to extract the precious building stone and slate. That, in turn, was sold off to the highest bidders.

Many of the properties were turned into country homes by outside buyers or turned into barns and stables. Valuables were melted down or smashed, statues of saints and other relics were destroyed or sold. Soon the great monasteries and almshouses had been reduced to nothing but ruins. St. Leonard's of York and St Mary of Bishopsgate, both large hospitals housing almost 200 patients, had nothing left to show for it. Glastonbury,

Shaftesbury, and Walsingham were obliterated. Henry VIII's reformation took away so much of the history of England's hospitals, including books and bibles, which were simply torn up. These religious institutions had constructed the foundation of purpose in caring for people. Yet, over 800 institutions had been wiped out and dramatically changed the social dynamic of the country forever.

Chapter Nine

A Culture of Death

The Middle Ages were abundant in the culture of death. Whether it was an execution in the town square or if you died a natural death, passing through to the next life was something medieval folks were passionate about. With high rates of mortality, be it by disease, famine, or war, death was a part of everyday life. The purpose of a good Christian life was to prepare for death. In the hopes that you would be accepted into God's kingdom, one would avoid sin by doing good works, being sure you kept up with the holy sacraments and the teachings of the Church. For the Church taught that salvation of your soul would entirely depend on your behaviour while on earth. As well, your death, which most times you could not control, was a determining factor in your passage to the next world. One always hoped for a good end, one that was in the comfort of your bed surrounded by your family, with the blessing of the priest bestowed upon you. It would be terrifying for all to have a sudden death and one that took you without the promise of confession. The Church taught that your confession assured your time in purgatory would be short. And you were sure to avoid hell, as long as you hadn't committed a mortal sin. The idea of purgatory in the Middle Ages was a genuine thing and entirely accepted as a teaching of the Church.

A part of the history of the Middle Ages is the practice of torture and execution but if we are to take a closer look at the actual timeline, very little of the offences took place between 500 and 1500. While the early through the mid-1500s are said to be after the medieval period, it appears this was when more of the infamous torture actually took place.

Yet, there is one case of torture that does stand out during the Middle Ages; the Knights Templar. The origins of the Knights Templar begin in the mid-twelfth century when a large organization of devout Christians set to carry out a mission. They were going to protect those on pilgrimage to the Holy Land. With formal endorsements from the Church, the group was subject to a papal bull issued in 1139. The Knights Templar no longer had to pay taxes and were held to no other authority than that of the Pope. The organisation quickly spread throughout Europe and gained financial influence, essentially becoming the first medieval banking system. Those going on pilgrimage could deposit their assets with the Templars in their home country. Upon arriving in Jerusalem, they could withdraw their funds from another branch of the Templars.

The Templars also became defenders of the Crusader states and earned a reputation as being battle-hardened fighters. As the Templars accrued significant amounts of assets and their power continued to spread throughout Europe, secular and religious leaders became increasingly critical of their wealth. It was King Philip IV of France who wanted to bring them down. Philip had led France to bankruptcy with the exhaustion of war and was desperate for any source of money that he came across. After killing two Popes and banishing all the Jews from France, Philip decided that the Templars were next.

On Friday, 13 October 1307, mass numbers of French Templars were arrested, including their Grand Master, Jacques de Molay. They were falsely accused of heresy, financial corruption, devil worship, and homosexuality. The king's instructions were as follows:

> You are to promise them pardon and favour if they confess the truth. But if not, you are to acquaint them that they will be condemned to death.

The purpose of torturing the Templars was not to reveal the truth; it was to obtain the truth that the accusers wanted to hear. In all, 138 Knight's Templars were tortured under King Philip, and most of them eventually confessed to crimes they did not commit. One of the most commonly used methods of torture used was Fire Torture. The victim's legs would be fastened in an iron frame and the soles of their feet smeared with fat or butter. They were then placed before a large fire where a screen was drawn backwards and forwards as if to moderate and regulate the heat of the flames. The pain inflicted by what was essentially roasting them alive caused the victims to confess in the hopes that the torture would stop. Starvation and sleep deprivation was also used, along with strappado, a device that:

> yanked the victim's tethered arms behind him until he was raised from the ground and his shoulders dislocated.

It is still interesting to think that these atrocities were growing in practice in the name of European monarchies. It is hard for us to imagine such things being done, even in countries where they still happen. But even though medieval times come to mind when the topic of inflicting pain becomes a discussion, we need to acknowledge that it was more than likely after the true Middle Ages. Torture was used as a means to extract a confession or to obtain the names of those that were guilty or could give the monarch information about crimes. The laws of the kingdom had no limit on the amount of torture that could be inflicted upon someone. The hope of getting a fair trial was limited, and often confessions were not taken seriously. The methods of torture used would depend on your crime, social ranking, and how greatly you had offended the king. Gender was also a consideration; however, depending on the monarch, even that could be overlooked.

The Tower of London had always been synonymous with torture, although it was only during the sixteenth and seventeenth centuries that it was used this way. Built shortly after the Norman Conquest, the Tower was constructed as a fortress to protect London, not a place to hold criminals and administer torture. However, the reputation the Tower has today is reflective of the practices carried out during the sixteenth and seventeenth centuries.

The rack was the most widely used method of torture in the Tower, as in the case of Anne Askew, who was condemned as a heretic in 1546. It was designed to expand the victim's body, dislocating the limbs from the socket. As in the case of Askew, the prisoner would be shown the rack in the hopes that they would provide answers to the questions of their interrogators. It was during the religious upheaval caused by the Reformation that the rack was primarily used.

Interestingly enough, it was Henry VIII and his two daughters, Queen Mary I and Queen Elizabeth I, who seemed to favour the device. Skeffington's Irons were also used during the reign of the Tudor king, although it isn't mentioned a lot in the Tower documents, so it is assumed it wasn't used as often as its sister method. Like the rack, Skeffington Irons were used to put tremendous pressure on the joints of the body. The idea was to hold your body in an uncomfortable position for an extremely long time. You would soon be overcome with such excruciating muscle cramps throughout your chest, neck, and limbs that you were almost sure to go mad. The body was compressed together rather than stretched apart.

One of the most horrifying methods of torture ever used was simply a rat and a cage. For many, the rat causes a sense of disgust in and by itself. A rat, usually one that was starved, was placed on the abdomen of the restrained victim. A cage with hot coals on the top was seated over the animal. In an attempt to escape the burning heat of the coals, the rat knew only one way out; through the stomach of the victim. It was an excruciating and slow method of torture as the rat had to use its claws and teeth to tear away at the flesh of the convicted. While this particular method was most often used during the Dutch Revolt, the use of rats as a means of torture was popular at the Tower of London during the reign of Elizabeth I. In a less sophisticated manner, rats were used in the blackened cells of the Tower that sat underneath the River Thames. Rats that were swept up from the rising river would tear away at the flesh of those imprisoned in the cells. Other methods included locking a prisoner in a space with a cluster of rats. It was hoped that the prisoner would slowly go mad from the rats gnawing at their body.

So many torture devices have been romanticised to fit the medieval era, such as the Pear of Anguish, the Catherine Wheel, the Iron Maiden (which didn't actually exist but was rather an eighteenth century legend), or the Head Crusher, to name a few. But most of these devices followed in the Elizabethan era rather than medieval times. This is certainly not to say that torture was nonexistent in the Middle Ages because it most certainly was, as was proven with the Knight's Templars. But the sophisticated methods of the later sixteenth and seventeenth century were not a part of it.

Executions, on the other hand, were something that was used quite frequently during the Middle Ages, and some of those methods were dreadful. It's important to understand that medieval executions were not merely there to entertain a bloodthirsty crowd. They were a complicated ordeal that has made the Middle Ages stand out. A person could be executed for several reasons, be it a crime against the people, a sin against God, or worse, high treason. Most executions were for the true criminal, who would usually have a traitor's death inflicted upon them. Crimes during the Middle Ages were taken seriously because they were atrocities committed against the very pillar of society. So much of the culture during medieval Europe was embedded in Christianity, and one's execution was viewed as punishment against the crimes that offended God. Executions were seen as a way of ensuring that a person met their death in a more timely fashion so that the Almighty might judge them. Every victim of execution was given a chance to confess their sins in the hopes that they would be saved from the gates of Hell.

In the case of the Grand Master of the Templars, de Molay, along with three other Templar leaders, were put on public display outside Notre Dame Cathedral. Three cardinals appointed by the Pope condemned them to life in prison. But King Philip wasn't satisfied with this and ordered both de Molay and his fellow leaders to be burned at the stake. Of the account in March 1314, historian Henry Charles Lea writes:

> That same day, by sunset, a pyre was erected on a small island in the Seine, the Ile des Juifs, near the palace garden. There de Molay, de Charney, de Gonneville, and de Peraud were slowly burned to death, refusing all offers of pardon for retraction, and bearing their torment with a composure which won for them the reputations of martyrs among the people, who reverently collected their ashes as relics.

The city of London is often associated with public executions. And with good measure. One of the most read about execution sites was Tyburn. Often referred to as "The Elms" because of the elm trees that flourished at the site, Tyburn was well known for its gallows during the Tudor era and thereafter. The gallows sported a wooden triangle arrangement known as the Three-Legged Mare. They were used for mass executions as several criminals could be hung at once. Being hung, although it was a quick death, was still horrific when considering the details. After your fall at the end of the noose, your cervical vertebrae, along with your spine, was ruptured. Your death came from compression of the arteries that supply blood to the head. It was hopeful that you would lose consciousness in only a few seconds, and your ultimate death would follow in the next five minutes or so. The methods of execution at Tyburn were intensely cruel. The first recorded execution was in 1196. William Fitz Osbert was a London citizen who played a significant role in the advocation of the poor as well as an 1196 uprising. He was stripped naked and dragged behind a horse to Tyburn. It was there that he was hanged.

It was in 1241 that the first death by drawing and quartering at Tyburn took place. Being drawn and quartered was if not one of, the most gruesome ways to be executed. Saved for the offenders that were convicted of high treason, you were:

> dragged upon a hurdle to the place of the execution, and then you shall be hanged by the neck and cut down while still alive. Your privy members were to be cut off, and your entrails to be taken out of your body and burned before your eyes. Your head will be then be cut off, your body to be divided into four quarters, and your head and quarters to be disposed of at the pleasure of the King's majesty.

The head of the executed was sometimes put on a pike for all to see at the Tower of London. We can only hope that almost everyone who had to endure such a cruel punishment fainted from the pain well before the worst of the execution took place. Scottish rebel William Wallace (1270–1305) was drawn and quartered at what was called The Elms, possibly either Tyburn or Smithfield, which was another execution site in London. Wallace faithfully led his country's revolt against England in a march towards freedom. In 1296, English King Edward I forced Scotland's monarch from his throne and claimed it for his own. Wallace was responsible for organising a Scottish uprising against the English. With his men, he invaded Northern England, and when he returned to Scotland in December 1297, he was knighted and proclaimed the guardian of the kingdom. His success was brief, however, because King Edward invaded Scotland and Wallace's troops suffered defeat. Wallace was captured and arrested near Glasgow and taken to England for trial. He was convicted of treason and taken to the Tower of London. There he was stripped of his clothing and dragged by a horse to the Elms. It was there that he was hung, drawn, and quartered. Like many others, his head was placed on a pike atop London Bridge. Thomas Culpepper (1514–1541), a courtier to Henry VIII, was found guilty of having an affair with Queen Katherine. At the time of the marriage, Henry was obese and ageing, and Queen Katherine was his beautiful teenage bride. Culpepper was in his twenties and extraordinarily handsome, and Queen Katherine was said to be very much in love with him, according to a letter kept in the National Archives. Though there is no actual proof that Katherine committed adultery, she became the victim as her cousin, Anne Boleyn, had. Her supposed lover, Culpepper, was initially sentenced to be drawn and quartered at Tyburn. Perhaps because of his devoted attention to the king that made him one of Henry's favourite courtiers, he was saved from this fate in the end. For the king showed him mercy and commuted the sentence to beheading. Francis Dereham (1513–1541), however, was not so lucky. Dereham is said to have taken Katherine's virginity before she came to court and married the king. Dereham had been appointed as a secretary at Hampton Court, and the news of his past affair with the queen caught the ear of the king's Privy Council. Dereham was executed along with Thomas Culpepper but the king did not show him the same mercy. He was drawn and quartered, and both men had their heads displayed at Tower Bridge.

Although executions were taken seriously in the medieval period, there surely were times when it became somewhat of a spectator sport. This was especially true of the Tyburn gallows, where it wasn't uncommon to see crowds gather to witness the executions of those who were sentenced to be hung. Roger Mortimer, 3rd Baron Mortimer, 1st Earl of March (1287–1330), was hung at Tyburn for his crimes against King Edward II. Along with his Queen Consort, Isabella, he led an invasion and rebellion against the king. Mortimer was eventually captured by the king's eldest son, Edward III, and sentenced to hanging. Although Isabella pleaded for Edward III to have mercy on Mortimer, it was to no avail. He was taken to Tyburn in November 1330 and hung. His dead body swung from the gallows for two days and two nights for everyone to witness. Perkin Warbeck (1474–1499), a pretender to the English throne, was also hung at Tyburn. Proclaiming he was Richard of Shrewsbury, Duke of York, he claimed a right to the crown and gained supporters. Warbeck was a threat to the reign of Henry VII. While Warbeck made landings in England backed by his small army, he was met with overwhelming resistance from Henry's men. He was held prisoner by Henry Tudor but treated very well during his captivity. After several failed attempts to escape, he was led from the Tower to Tyburn in November 1499, where he was hung for treason.

In 1401, under the reign of King Henry VI of England, *De heretic comburendo* (Regarding the Burning of Heretics) was passed into law. The law declared that those with false and perverse heretic beliefs should renounce their views, or they would "be burnt, that such punishment may strike fear into the minds of others".

Bayfield was taken to Smithfield in December 1531 and set on fire at the stake. Records show that he suffered greatly as the fire didn't consume him immediately. He continued in prayer until he was engulfed and died.

Although Henry VIII had transformed the religion of England, Catholicism would make a comeback under the reign of his daughter, Mary I. Though her reign far reaches that of the medieval era, I feel it is important to mention her, as she is notorious in English history for her demeanour. Mary was a fervent Catholic and had pledged that she would return the country to what she deemed the true faith. Under her rule, any Protestant who did not convert or tried to flee the county would risk being burned. It is estimated that over 300 Protestants died because of their faith during her reign. Smithfield Market would become synonymous with the burnings she ordered. The executions earned her the title *Bloody Mary*. The convicted prisoner would have stood in an empty tar barrel, with stocks of wood piled around them. Death by burning was a prolonged and painful ordeal and the smell of burnt flesh was said to have lingered continuously at Smithfield during the consistent burnings

Death by burning at the stake has been part of history in several cultures and a portion of Europe during medieval times. In the Kingdom of Aragon in 1197, Peter II (1178–1213) made burning for heretics law. The Holy Roman Emperor, Fredrick II (1194–1250), made burning legal by statute in 1231 in Italy, and in France, it became law in 1270 under Louis IX. With the intent of safeguarding the Catholic faith, the Spanish Inquisition was established in 1478 under the rule of King Ferdinand and Queen Isabella. Under the order of execution by burning, it is estimated that roughly 2000 people lost their lives between 1478 and 1490 alone.

Throughout most of history, Jews have been the subject of blame and persecution. During much of the Middle Ages in Europe, they were denied citizenship along with the rights it would have assured them. In 1096, during the First Crusade, a wave of antisemitism swept over France and Italy. Through the fifteenth century and beyond, this hatred continued. Only Jews who had converted to Christianity were tolerated, and many faced mass expulsions. In 1348, a Jewish man named Bona was executed most ruthlessly. The Breaking Wheel, or Catherine Wheel, was a method of torture and public execution that had been used as far back as the eighth century BCE. Those convicted and sentenced to execution were taken to a public scaffold where they would be "broken by the wheel". The Execution Wheel was a sizeable wooden spoke wheel, much like those used on carts and litters. The goal of the wheel was to inflict mutilation before execution. The accused was first strapped down to the ground. The wheel, which was almost always made of dense wood, was then dropped on top of them. The executioner would start at the shin bones and continue to drop the wheel as he worked his way up the body. A second wooden wheel was introduced, and the accused's broken body was thread through the spokes on the wheel. The wheel was set upon a pole, and it was up to the executioner if the victim were to be strangled or decapitated. Sometimes a fire was set up underneath them. It was then that they were simply left for dead to the delight of scavenging animals. The Jewish man Bona remained conscious for four days after being left to rot on the wheel after his punishment. Jews were not only blamed for the death of Christ, but as the Black Death raged on in the mid-fourteenth century, they were blamed for that as well. Well-established Jewish communities were demolished, and their inhabitants burned. In February 1349, in the city of Strasbourg in France, hundreds of Jews were publicly burned to death in retaliation against the Black Death.

Beheading remains one of the most talked-about forms of execution, and it's been in practice for over 5000 years at least. Civilizations throughout time have used decapitation as a form of punishment, and in some cultures, it was considered an honourable way to go. It was a quick and relatively painless death, as long as the executioner's axe was sharp and his aim true. Almost every monarchy England has had has at least one beheading documented.

Sadly, throughout Western Europe, there remain several detailed accounts of beheadings that didn't go smoothly. England alone is accountable for more than one execution that didn't go as planned, and I feel they are worth mention.

In the case of Thomas Cromwell, his execution was an atrocity. Cromwell faithfully served Henry VIII for almost ten years and he was an avid supporter of the Reformation. He lost the king's affections after arranging a marriage to the German princess, Anne of Cleves. Although Cromwell was hopeful for this marriage, the king was not pleased with Cromwell's choice. The king claimed he could not be aroused by her, thus keeping him from producing another son. Cromwell was executed for both treason and heresy in July 1540. There are witnesses during his execution that claim the headsman was still drunk from the previous night out at a pub and had great difficulty swinging his axe. There is mention that Cromwell was initially hit in the shoulder blades more than once before his head was successfully removed. It was later in his reign that Henry VIII expressed great regret for the punishment he bestowed upon Cromwell. Margaret Pole, Countess of Salisbury (1473–1541), daughter of the Duke of Clarence, Edward IV's brother, and one of the few remaining family members of the Plantagenets. Despite being governess to his daughter Mary, Henry VIII had her executed not long after Cromwell. She was accused of supporting Catholicism and being a traitor. She was given no trial yet went to her execution with dignity at the age of 67. Several rumours claim that she ran from the headsman upon entering the scaffold, but many historians claim this is largely falsified. Sadly her execution was not carried out swiftly. Eustace Chapuys, ambassador to the Holy Roman Empire, was present at her execution and wrote that the executioner had been a "wretched and blundering youth who literally hacked her head and shoulders to pieces in the most pitiful manner".

This leads me to discuss whether or not death is immediate at the time of decapitation and to touch upon stories such as what happened to Mary Queen of Scots after her execution, whose lips were said to "have stirred up and down a quarter of an hour after her head was cut off". Unconsciousness will occur within a few seconds after the brain is deprived of oxygen. Although some suggest that there remains a period of consciousness after decapitation, most modern doctors agree that it is more than likely a reflexive twitch of the face muscles rather than an intentional movement. It would be wise to assume that following the loss of blood, the condemned is not able to perceive pain.

While it is hard to estimate genuinely, it has been perceived that Henry VIII ordered over 50,000 executions during his thirty-seven year reign. A significant number of them were beheadings, including two of his wives, whose stories have become infamous throughout history. Arguably the most famous execution in English history, if not certainly during the reign of Henry VIII, is the execution of Queen Anne Boleyn. I've gone into a bit of detail regarding her execution, though it was roughly thirty years after the medieval period. Her execution is one of the most notorious in history, and I feel she is worthy of mention.

Anne was the second wife of the king and a prominent reformer. While married to his first wife, Henry's obsession with Anne began in early 1526 when she secured a post as a lady-in-waiting to the current queen. With Anne's promise of a son, Henry divorced his first wife and changed the face of English history with the Reformation. His desire for Anne completely clouded his reason, and they were married in January 1533. Anne would give Henry another heir but not the son he so desired. After several miscarriages, Henry grew frustrated with his queen and soon found a reason to be rid of her as well. He had Anne investigated in April 1536 for acts of treason and infidelity. She was arrested and sent to the Tower of London, along with her brother, George Boleyn (1503–1536), and several other of her "lovers".

Along with the others, Anne was sentenced to die. However, in a last show of mercy, Henry hired an expert swordsman from France to perform her execution rather than have a queen beheaded with an axe. William Kingston (1476–1540), the Constable of the Tower, was with the queen for the last few days of her life. On the morning of her execution, he wrote:

> This morning she sent for me, that I might be with her at such time as she received the good Lord, to the intent I should hear her speak as touching her innocence away to be clear. And in the writing of this she sent for me, and at my coming said, 'Mr. Kingston, I hear I shall not die before noon, and I am very sorry therefore, for I thought to be dead by this time and past my pain.'

The queen's execution had been delayed a day, and one can imagine the trepidation she must have felt. She had prepared herself for her death, only to hear it was postponed. Kingston went on to write:

> And then she said, 'I heard say the executioner was very good, and I have a little neck.' And then put her hands about it, laughing heartily. I have seen many men and also women executed, and that they have been in great sorrow, and to my knowledge, this lady has much joy in death.

On the morning of 19 May 1536, Anne Boleyn climbed the scaffold on the north side of the White Tower, accompanied by her ladies. Like the queen that would follow her less than ten years later, Anne held her head high with dignity. Her short speech to the crowd is as follows:

Good Christian people, I am come hitherto die, for according to the law, and by the law, I am judged to die, and therefore I will speak nothing against it. I am come hither to accuse no man, nor to speak anything of that, whereof I am accused and condemned to die, but I pray God save the King and send him long to reign over you, for a gentler nor a more merciful prince was there never. And to me, he was ever a good, a gentle and sovereign Lord. And if any person will meddle of my cause, I require them to judge the best. And thus, I take my leave of the world and of you all, and I heartily desire you all to pray for me. O Lord have mercy on me, to God, I commend my soul.

And by command of the king, Queen Anne Boleyn was executed with one swipe of the executioner's sword.

Anne Boleyn was among the lucky ones who received the mercy of the monarchy when it came to beheadings. The executioner's tool was usually the bearded axe, as this was a weapon commonly used in England. In Britain, beheading was used by the Anglo Saxons and it was brought back after the Battle of Hastings. It was most often used for those of noble birth who had been convicted of high treason. It is impossible to name everyone who was beheaded in England alone as it would take up pages upon pages. However, a few that deserve mention are Thomas, 2nd Earl of Lancaster (1278–1322), who was beheaded under Edward II, and Thomas de Mowbray, 4th Earl of Norfolk (1385–1405), who was beheaded under Henry IV for treason. Sir Owen Tudor (1400–1461) was executed by Edward IV for being a Lancastrian, and Sir Thomas More was beheaded by Henry VIII for refusing to sign the Oath of Supremacy. The beheadings in France don't compare to the number of those in England until the Reign of Terror. More specifically, when the guillotine was invented in 1789 as a means to a more merciful death. In Scotland, several people were executed for their rebellion against the king. Walter Stewart, Earl of Atholl, Strathearn, and Caithness (1360–1437) was a Scottish Noble who was sentenced to beheading after he conspired to murder James I. John Douglas, Lord of Balvenie (1433–1463), the youngest of the five Black Douglas Brothers, was beheaded for his rebellion against King James II (1430–1460). In Spain, a number of people were beheaded in 1135 under the reign of Ramiro II (1086–1157), King of Aragon, for the act of treason.

Society in the Middle Ages was surrounded by what I call a culture of death. Death was always close at hand, a regular, if unwelcome visitor in the everyday lives of both rich and poor. It made no resolve regarding your social status and cared nothing for your means of wealth. While the rich may have been able to afford what was deemed as better medical care, in the end, it didn't matter once it was your time. A constant source of grief in the Middle Ages was the death of small children and babies that lived but a few hours. This was an unfortunate part of life that, sadly, many parents had to face. But just because it was more common than today, their grief at such a loss was genuine. Even the highest-ranking members of society experienced sorrow as a whole. It was especially hard for a member of royalty to lose an heir as it caused problems in the line of succession. Grand festivities were put into the celebration of a son and heir, and to have the loss of such a person caused great sadness.

Edward of Middleham (1473–1484), the only son of Richard III, was especially important to the throne as he was the one promise to the succession that Richard had. Richard had seized the throne from his late brother Edward IV, after declaring that his children were not legitimate, so the safety of his own heir was crucial. But Edward was not a healthy child and was mostly kept away from the public. Despite a grand ceremony pronouncing him as Prince of Wales, he died of tuberculosis less than one year later. He was only ten years old. The Croyland Chronicle, a historical chronicle from the fifteenth century, states:

> the only son of his, in whom all the hopes of the royal succession, fortified with so many oaths, were centered, was seized with an illness of but short duration, and died at Middleham Castle, in the year of our Lord, 1484, being the first of the reign of the said King Richard. On hearing the news of this, at Nottingham, where they were residing, you might have seen his father and mother in a state of almost bordering on madness, by reason of their sudden grief.

Henry, Duke of Cornwall, being the heir apparent of Henry VIII, was an especially devastating loss to the monarchy. The king and queen had already lost a child, who was stillborn at birth. Henry VIII was especially concerned about having a surviving heir to the throne, and he was consumed with carrying on the Tudor line. His older brother, Arthur, had been heir apparent to the throne when he died of what was believed to have been the sweating sickness. It was essential to have an "heir and a spare" if something happened to the heir. When Henry's son, the Duke of Cornwall, was born on the first of January 1511, a lavish and extravagant affair was held in the child's honour. The prince was loved immeasurably by his father along with the court, but sadly he was taken from them six weeks later. It is not known exactly what caused the death of the child but reports state that both parents were understandably hysterical at the loss of their future king. Queen Katherine would give birth to two more children who died under three months of age before their only living child, a girl, was born in 1516. A further pregnancy in 1518 would result in stillbirth.

Grief as a whole was prevalent not only in the loss of children but of spouses. William I of England was described as "weeping most profusely for days" at the death of his wife and queen, Matilda of Flanders. After the death of his beloved Queen Jane, who gave him the heir he so desired, Henry VIII is said to have locked himself away at Windsor Castle. The king had spent hours by her bedside in distress when it was clear she would die. His mourning went on for months, and he refused to see anyone while he wallowed in his misery.

Interestingly enough, demonstrations of grief by men were not viewed favourably in other countries. Looked at as being unmanly, during the thirteenth and fourteenth centuries in several communities in Italy, it was actually banned. Emotional outbursts were forbidden and would be punished accordingly. It was acceptable to shed a few tears, but any hollering or wailing was not. Throughout Europe, it was undoubtedly more acceptable for a woman to show such emotion as they were looked at as naturally overly emotional, and perhaps it was expected of them.

With the constant threat of death everywhere, especially during plague outbreaks, much of medieval life was spent preparing for it. Death was looked at more as a doorway to everlasting life. It was a transition of the soul into the next world. The culture of the Middle Ages was more about how you lived your life in preparation for death. And like almost everything in medieval times, death was shaped entirely by the Catholic Church. While they taught that the soul was eternal, you would be judged accordingly for your actions before being accepted into the Kingdom of Heaven. The reminder of death was consistent throughout the Middle Ages in the form of art and literature. Especially in the years following the

Black Death, there was a massive trend in art that emphasised death rather than turning away from it. Images of corpses were almost everywhere, especially on tombs. The image of death coming for reluctant individuals was common. The constant reminder of death was also prevalent in the images of demons at deathbed scenes. They seemed to be always ready to snag you away to hell. Dancing skeletons, even though in a merry mood, appeared to remind you that death was everywhere. *The Danse Macabre*, from the mid-fifteenth century, was an image that was popular after the Black Death. Dancing skeletons are seen leading people to dance, rich and poor. This image represented the idea that one was absolutely powerless in the face of death.

During the twelfth century, the Church claimed that all who died would undergo the process of purification known as Purgatory. Purgatory was a chance for those who had died to atone for their sins and it was made official by Pope Innocent IV (1195–1254) in 1254. Purgatory was a place of darkness and terror that all souls had to pass through. One's time in the fire-filled world was comparable to their sins. In other words, the punishment fit the crime. Purgatory may have been a place of pain and torture, but it wasn't permanent. The best defence against a long time spent here was to be good in life, for one's social status in Purgatory mattered not. During life, it was important to invest in one's salvation through the means of almsgiving and donations to the poor. It was also imperative that Mass was attended regularly as these things were all thought to lessen the time in Purgatory. And when your death was near, one looked to the afterlife. Before departing, one was given a chance to redeem themselves for any wrongdoings. With the presence of clergy at the death bed, it was important to make confessions in the last moments on earth. Prayer for amends was part of the culture of death in the Middle Ages and a vital ritual to ease one's transgression.

Along with the importance of the Eucharist, a priest at the bedside was central in consoling the dying. The prayers of a priest, as well as the anointing of oil, offered great comfort. It was believed that if one confessed while receiving their last rights, they were to be forgiven.

The Catholic Church had a strict set of rules that were intended to be followed regarding funerals, as the passage from the land of the living to the realm of the dead was a frightening time. Not only for those passing through but for loved ones saying goodbye as well. Rites of the Church ensured that the departed would be comfortable on their journey. The funeral procession was an essential part of one's passage and it was a very public display of the family's wealth or lack thereof. The grander the funeral, the better. Large groups of mourners, along with the ringing of the church bells, spoke volumes regarding one's status. Candles and torches lit to honour the dead were also crucial in marking one's social status. The place of burial was also vital, and those with elite status, even clerics, were buried in the Church near the altar.

The extravagance of a funeral in Medieval Europe wholly depended on your rank in the feudal world. One could expect a simple pauper's burial, which would have been similar to the burial rituals of a leper, or if you were of higher rank, an elaborate funeral on a grand scale could be had. Much of it also depended on what the family was willing to do.

For a well-to-do merchant or tradesman, the body would be washed and shrouded before it would lie in state. Perhaps this would happen at the home of the deceased or in a church. Though this was not a formal viewing period, those who wished to see the body could do so. A Mass would have been said for the soul of the deceased, and the more money the family donated to the Church, the more prayers they could expect. A large meal would have been laid out after the burial where family and friends would have been served meat.

The poor played an important role in the funerals of others during the Middle Ages. The widows, orphans, blind and those with disabilities became the mourners. The prayers of the poor and sick were thought to be quite commendable. The poor would receive a new robe, along with cheese and bread for their service to the family of the deceased.

If you were poor and employed by a respectable family, they would usually pay for the funeral. But to a much smaller degree, such as having one's name included in a Mass instead of a Mass being said for them. There would be a simple burial in the churchyard with no elaborate funeral to mark the occasion.

The death of a monarch or noble would have been on a much grander scale than any commoner could expect. The death of Elizabeth of York, queen of King Henry VII, was an unpleasant shock to both her husband and England. The king ordered no expense spared at her funeral. On her death, church bells throughout London rang in her honour. Her body was washed and dressed in beautiful robes and her children were brought to say goodbye to their mother. Her embalming took place on that same day. The ancient practice of embalming, which began in Ancient Egyptian culture, spread to Europe in about 500 CE. During the Middle Ages, the process involved the removal of the organs, cleansing the body with alcohol, and inserting herbs into previously made incisions.

During the Renaissance, new techniques were being used for embalming fluids. In the studies of Leonardo da Vinci (1452–1519), his embalming fluids consisted of turpentine, lavender oil, camphor, wine, vermillion, and rosin. Embalming was mainly for the rich as it required great skill, and expensive materials were needed. After her embalming, the queen's body was rubbed with spices and sweet wine and wrapped in a waxed cloth. Her body was then encased in lead and placed in a coffin covered in velvet and damask.

The coffin was carried under a canopy to the Chapel of St. Peter in the Tower of London. The walls of the chapel were draped in black cloth, and 500 candles burned for her. The queen's body lay in state under the watchful eye of her ladies. For three days, Masses were said along with the Lord's Prayer. On the day of her funeral, 22 February 1503, after a Mass, her coffin was placed on a carriage. The carriage had been lined with blue cloth of gold and black velvet and was drawn by six elegant horses draped in velvet. A beautiful lifelike effigy that wore the robes of estate was placed on top of her coffin. There was great detail in her long hair, and her fingers were alive with precious stones and gold. Her procession to Westminster Abbey was watched by mourners who lined the streets to say goodbye to their queen. Next to the carriage rode knights that followed the hundreds of poor who led the procession. Her ladies rode behind the carriage on their own horses dressed in black velvet. A gentleman dressed in black led the carriage. The queen's casket lay in state at Westminster the night before the funeral. And on that day, candles were lit, and an impressive display of her coat of arms was in constant view. The Bishop of Lincoln officiated at the funeral Mass, and the Bishop of Rochester gave her sermon. Her grave was blessed before her coffin was placed amid a flow of tears from onlookers. It is estimated that the equivalent the king spent on her funeral would amount to more than a million pounds today.

In addition to showing her rank as queen, a big funeral would have meant a good start to things in Purgatory for Elizabeth. The Church believed that one physically experienced Purgatory, so one needed enough support to go through such an ordeal. Spiritual assistance to the dead, in the form of prayer and masses, was often put in a person's will before they passed. It was believed that the more extravagance that was put into your funeral would assure you a reduced time in Purgatory. The more money that was left to the Church meant the more you would be prayed for after your death. A Catholic Mass was the best thing for you, and the wealthier you were, the more you could afford. In the cases of kings and queens, money was often spent to ensure that a Mass was said for you well into the afterlife. Henry VII's death was paid for not only with money but with the promise of tens of thousands of Masses to be said until the end of time. It was also vital that you were charitable in your life, as this was another thing that would ensure you found your way to Heaven. Charity through hospitals and giving to the poor would ensure that you were prayed for by those to whom you had given. As Masses were pertinent at almshouses, having groups of people pray for you was essential.

Of course, not all funerals went off as flawless as Elizabeth of York's. Especially because embalming techniques were primitive, the muddled aftermath of a monarch's burial, or anyone's for that matter, was not unheard of. In the cases of kings, some were well documented.

William the Conqueror will always be known as the victor at the Battle of Hastings in 1066. But this new King of England would meet a rather inglorious end. Though he did establish social reform throughout England, along with forging ties with France and building some of the most impressive structures known to man, William was also a martinet. His occupation of England had developed into a form of military dictatorship, with the country divided into areas assigned by military governors. In 1069, in what was known as "the Harrying of the North", William and his men seized land by burning down villages and crops. Women, along with the farm animals, were slaughtered or reportedly reduced to cannibalism. Afterwards William indulged in food and drink for the next twenty years. In 1087, his massive bulk most likely contributed to his end. William was in France with his son Robert when his horse spooked, much to his shock. The animal is said to have reared up aggressively, and the pommel on the saddle injured William. The horse had jerked up with such force that the pommel punctured the king's stomach. With what was most likely infection from the saddle introduced to his intestines, the king spent the next six weeks slowly dying. Perhaps this gave him time to think about his salvation, as he was said to have made a credible deathbed confession. While the historical reports are a bit skewed, there seems to be no doubt that he was sincere over what he had done in life. In the historical chronicles of Orderic Vitalis (1075–1142), an oblate who had spent his childhood at the abbey of Saint Evroul in the Duchy of Normandy, the king had confessed with these words:

> I treated the native inhabitants of the kingdom with reasonable severity, cruelly oppressed high and low, unjustly disinherited many, and caused the death of thousands by starvation and war, especially in Yorkshire. In mad fury, I descended on the English of the North like a raging lion and ordered that their homes and crops with all their equipment and furnishing should be burnt at once and their great flocks and herds of sheep and cattle slaughtered everywhere. So, I chastised a great multitude of men and women with the lash of starvation and, alas! was the cruel murderer of many thousands, both young and old, of this fair people.

It should be known that while Vitalis is listed as a credible source, many historians question if this exact speech was William's. Some claim that the statement was more of an interpretation of what Vitalis would have liked to have heard, and perhaps he thought to give praise to the dying king by claiming such words passed his lips. But it is clear that on his deathbed, William the Conqueror did show regret and was believed to have made a good end to his life. On 9 September 1087, when the king finally succumbed to his injuries, he was all but abandoned by his men. Vitalis writes:

> The lesser attendants, seeing that their supporters had absconded, seized the arms, vessels, clothing, linen, and all the royal furnishings, and hurried away leaving the King's body almost naked on the floor of the house. They left him as if he had been a barbarian.

No one who had served the king had prepared for his burial. It was then that a knight of unknown origin was:

> induced by his natural goodness to undertake the charge of the funeral, for the love of God and honour of his country. He, therefore, procured at his own expense persons to embalm and carry the body.

The seventy mile trip to Caen, France, would wreak absolute havoc on the king's corpse. Bacteria from William's stomach had begun to leak out into the rest of his body. The tissue started to decompose at an accelerated rate, and an array of noxious gases began to emerge. To make matters worse, his funeral in Caen was delayed by a raging fire that consumed many of the mourners. The heat of the fire also caused William's body to inflate even more so that it no longer fit into his final resting place. In an attempt to lower his body, his men were shocked when "his swollen bowels burst, and an intolerable stench assailed the nostrils of the bystanders and the whole crowd". The overwhelming mess and, no doubt, the smell caused the funeral to be rushed through as everyone was desperate to get away from the offending stink.

A similar scenario went down with Henry VIII after his death on 28th January 1547. Almost two weeks after his death, his coffin began its procession to Windsor, the same resting place of his father and beloved queen, Jane Seymour. While the march in itself was something out of a fairy tale, with a horse-drawn chariot carrying the coffin through the streets, it was the aftermath of what happened to Henry's body that is most often remembered. Later in his life, the ageing king had become quite obese. It is said that he consumed around 5000 calories a day. Aside from his enormous girth, he weighed close to 400lbs. Henry was still plagued with painful, pus-filled boils on his legs. His jousting accident in 1536 had caused his existing leg wound to become bothersome again, to the point where his doctors found it very hard to treat. Both of these ailments prevented Henry from being the sportsman he had been in his younger days, and his sedentary condition only added to his weight. During the procession to Windsor, the deceased king and his entourage stopped overnight at Syon Abbey. It was witnessed that the king's corpse had begun to leak bodily fluids through cracks in the coffin. Although there is some speculation, it has been mentioned that one of the monks was present to see some of the abbey dogs lick the king's remains from the floor.

Whether or not these stories have been elaborated through time, we will never know for sure. There is certainly no doubt that the embalming methods and construction of the casket left a medieval corpse subject to further damage.

If one were a criminal and had been executed as such, they could look forward to not only a lengthy stay in Purgatory but that their remains would be given almost no respect. The bodies of criminals were often impaled, or their heads put on pikes and left to wild animals. Mutilation of a corpse often followed an execution of a criminal. Bodies were thrown into a well or fed to dogs or pigs. This treatment was almost expected as criminals were deemed useless and unfit to have even their remains treated with respect. Separate cemeteries were often made for the remains of criminals as they were considered to be so impure that they posed a threat to society.

There were certain burial practices that the Church viewed as cruel and banned. The German tradition of disembowelling the body, dismembering it, and cooking the flesh so that it came off of the bones made for more accessible transport of the body, especially if you were away from home. This practice was extremely important to dignitaries and was used into the thirteenth century. But in 1299, Pope Boniface VIII condemned the ritual, calling it a savage abuse and deemed it cruel. Although the Church warned that resurrection might be at risk by dismembering the body, this ban was often ignored by the elite.

Along with this, other burial rites of the Church were sometimes disregarded. In the thirteenth and fourteenth centuries, it was advised to remove a dead baby from the mother if both had died in childbirth. It was believed that the child still needed to be baptised, and the question arose as to whether the mother could be placed in consecrated ground. If she had not been churched after the birth or failure of, she was still considered unclean. Particularly in the later Middle Ages, this practice was also ignored by several. In rare cases, what was known as a coffin birth could arise after the mother had been buried with her child still in the womb. This type of postmortem birth was caused by the pressure of abdominal gases that would discharge the fetus after both mother and baby had been buried. While it is extremely rare today, embalming methods may not have been sophisticated enough during the Middle Ages to prevent this. While there have been documented cases in the sixteenth century of this happening, a discovery in 2010 revealed a coffin birth in the Italian town of Imola. Archaeologists discovered the skeleton of a pregnant woman believed to have died in the seventh or eighth century. They found a small gathering of fetal bones between her legs and determined that the baby must have been born postmortem at roughly thirty-eight weeks gestation. They also discovered a small hole in the mother's skull that presented in such a way that it was suggested that it was not done in a violent manner. According to archaeologists who studied the case, it was believed that the hole was drilled as part of the surgical procedure known as trepanation. While the surgery was performed during the Middle Ages for a plethora of reasons, the general theory in the case of this mother is that she may have been suffering from eclampsia. She may have been treated with trepanation in an attempt to save her, but judging from the wounds on the woman's skull, scientists believed that she died about one week after the procedure.

While folks in the Middle Ages dedicated much of their lives to preparing for the next, it was a terrifying ordeal to die a sudden death or one that you hadn't prepared well for. A "good death" was one at home, where loved ones and the priest surrounded the dying. Folks believed that your soul left your body at the moment of your death, and being sure that you had your salvation was of enormous significance. Because of the plague especially, mortality rates were very high. Epidemics caused utter panic as plans for one's burial were ruined, and you were at the mercy of death without salvation. The disarray caused by the Black Death had people believing it was the Apocalypse and a good end was almost impossible. The number of dead outweighed the number of priests, and they certainly weren't immune to the grasp of the plague. Piles upon piles of corpses were disposed of with no hope for a proper ceremony. Because the Church was against the idea of cremation, believing one could not be resurrected if cremated, newly consecrated ground known as plague cemeteries began to form to try to accommodate the thousands that died. As quoted by Boccaccio in his *Decameron*:

> Many breathed their last in the open street, whilst other many, for all they died in their houses, made it known to the neighbours that they were dead rather by the stench of their rotting bodies than otherwise; and of these and others who died all above the multitude of corpses aforesaid, which daily and nightly, hourly came carried in crowds to every church, especially if it were sought to give each his own place, according to ancient usance, there were made throughout the Churchyards, after every other part was full, vast trenches.

One's power and riches meant very little in the face of sudden death. The Black Death haunted the minds of everyone, and a constant state of anxiety flowed throughout Europe.

The second of November, deemed All Souls Day, was made official by Rome in the thirteenth century. This was a day to remember all the souls still in Purgatory through the Mass. All Souls Day became important because if you had died a sudden death or if you didn't have the riches to ensure you had a proper funeral, then your soul would be prayed for. During All Souls Day, it was especially important to tend to the poor in the hopes that the acts of service would help folks in Purgatory pass through to Heaven's gate. As with the lepers, Jesus believed that the poor were closer to God and they could help those around them with prayer.

A great deal of money had been given to the Church in asking for pardons and grand Masses that the Church soon became self-indulgent. In the mid-fifteenth century, early reformers started to take issue with these practices and demanded change. Reformers had a problem with the Church's belief in Purgatory and saw it as further evidence of their greed. They questioned why the Church was asking its people for money for Masses when Purgatory wasn't in scripture. It became referred to as a "vain imagination". In 1529, the English Parliament forbade the purchase of Masses for the dead. Reformers believed that the Church played upon the uncertainty of folks in the face of death when it came to their salvation. They stressed that "Christ had already defeated the powers of death, sin, and hell for mankind".

And they rejected the idea that the Catholic Church stood to make themselves richer by preying upon its people. This was only fuel for the fire in the case of the English Reformation. As this progressed, many Catholic traditions for death were denounced. Reformers rejected not only the idea of Purgatory but other death bed rituals, such as the presence of the clergy and masses to be said for the dead. Edward VI, son of Henry VIII, passed the dissolution of the chantry. He believed that a priest should not be compensated to say mass for those who had departed, and with his new law, they were more or less pushed from the new Church of England. Edward made great strides to further the Reformation his father had started and believed that his salvation came by his faith alone and not by the forgiveness of sins. He thought that Catholic rituals were of no help to anyone and deemed them more of a hindrance. Through his reign, Edward VI changed the face of death in England for years to come.

Notes and Sources

Chapter One
On the Theory of Humourism and the Hippocratic Corpus, look at *Galen and the Gateway to Medicine by* Jeanne Bendick.
On the Temple of Asclepius, look at *The Public Physicians of Ancient Greece* by Louis Cohn-Haft.
On the Sacred Disease, look at *Philosophy and Medicine in Ancient Greece* by WHS Jones.
On the Canon of Medicine, see *Ibn Arabi in the Later Islamic Tradition* by Alexander Knysh.
On the Zodiac Man, see *Discovery of the Zodiac Man in Cuneiform* by John Wee.

Chapter Two
On the Roman Empire, look at *Life, Death, and Entertainment in the Roman Empire* by David Stone Potter.
On Benedict of Nursia, see *Religion in the Middle Ages* by Simon Newman.
On Benedictine monks, see *Medieval Monastery* by Mark Cartwright.
On The Book of Hours, see *The Book of Hours* by John Harthan.
On demonic possession, look at *Medieval and Renaissance Depictions of Possession and Exorcism* by Meghan MacRae.

Chapter Three
On feudalism and plumbing, look at *The Time Traveler's Guide to Medieval England* by Ian Mortimer.
On castles, see *Life In a Medieval Castle* by J Gies.
On Erasmus, see *The English Reformation* by AG Dickens.
On groom of the stool, see *Royal Palaces of London* by S Thurley.
On children, see *Childhood in Anglo-Saxon England* by Sally Crawford and *Growing up in Medieval England* by Barbara Hanawalt.
On the homes of peasants, look at *A Tudor Housewife* by Alison Sim.

Chapter Four
On medieval towns, see *The Time Travelers Guide to Medieval England* by Ian Mortimer.
On smallpox, see *Armies of Pestilence* by RS Bray.
On the miasmic theory, see *A Brief History of the Miasmic Theory* by Carl Sterner.
On dysentery, see *The Conquest of Epidemic Disease* by Charles Winslow.

On syphilis, see *The Pox-The Life and Near Death of a Very Social Disease* by Kevin Brown.
On sweating sickness, see *Young Henry; The Rise of Henry VIII* by Robert Hutchinson and *The Sweating Sickness in Tudor England; a Plague of the Renaissance* by Philip Liebson.
On leprosy, see *Leprosy in Medieval England* by Carole Rawcliffe.
On the Black Death, see *Doctors of the Black Death* by Jackie Rosenjek, *The Black Death* by Paul Slade, *The Black Death and the Future of Medicine* by Sarah Venneste, *Children During the Black Death* by Shona Wray, *The Black Death* by Philip Ziegler, *Black Death; The Complete History* by Ole Benedicto, *Medical Sourcebook; The Decameron* by Giovanni Boccaccio, *Daily Life During the Black Death* by Joseph Byrne, *In the Wave of the Plague* by NF Cantor, *Behind the Mask; The Plague Doctor* by Dr Lindsey Fitzharris, *The Black Death* by RS Gottfried, and *The Great Mortality* by John Kelly.

Chapter Five
On childbed fever, see *The Trotula; An English Translation of the Medieval Compendium of Women's Medicine* by Monica Green, and *Medieval Royal Babies of England* by Cynthia Hyno.
On menstruation, see *A History of Jewish Gynaecological Texts in the Middle Ages* by Ron Barkai and *The Trotula; An English Translation of the Medieval Compendium of Women's Medicine* by Monica Green.
On the Trotula, Secreta Mulierune (Secrets of Women), and the formation of the foetus, see *The Trotula; An English Translation of the Medieval Compendium of Women's Medicine* by Monica Green.
On the formation of the foetus and signs of conception, see *Milestones in Midwifery and the Secret Instrument* by Walter Radcliff, *Birth Control in the West in the Thirteenth and Fourteenth Centuries* by PA Billier.
On Wellcome Apocalypse and The Disease Woman see *The Miracle of Childbirth; The Portrayal of Parturient Women in Medieval Miracle Narratives* by Hilary Powell, *The Trotula; An English Translation of the Medieval Compendium of Women's Medicine* by Monica Green.
On prayer amulets and pilgrimages see, *English People and Their Prayers* by Eamon Duffy and *Performance Rituals for Conception and Childbirth in England* by Peter Jones.
On the Sloane Manuscripts, look at *Medieval Woman's Guide to Health* by Beryl Rowland.
On royal children, look at *Medieval Royal Babies of England* by Cynthia Hyno.

Chapter Six
On John Gaddesden, see *Annals of the Royal College of Surgeons in England* by JJ Kirkpatrick.
On uroscopy, see *Urine Color; Symptoms and Causes*, and *Looking at Urine; Renaissance of an Unbroken Tradition* by Garabed Eknoyan.

Notes and Sources 191

On syphilis, Sive Morbus Gallicus, see *The Pox-The Life and Near Death of a Very Social Disease* by Kevin Brown.
On mercury treatment, see *Medieval and Early Renaissance Medicine* by Nancy Saraisi.
On the illnesses of Henry VIII, see *The Physical Decline of Henry VIII* by Sarah Bryson.
On sweating sickness, see *The Sweating Sickness in Tudor England; a Plague of the Renaissance* by Philip Liebson.
On John of Arderne see, *Medicine in the English Middle Ages* by Faye Getz, and *The Qualities and Conduct of an English Surgeon* by JJ Kirkpatrick.
On bloodletting see, *Medicine in the English Middle Ages* by Faye Getz and *Cutting Edge; Early History of the Surgeons of London* by Theodore Beck.
On cupping, see *The Face of Mercy* by Matthew Naythons.
On Al-Zahrawi, see *The House of Wisdom; How the Arabs Transformed Western Civilization* by Jonathan Lyons.
On Guy de Chauliac, see *Guy de Chauliac, The Father of Surgery* by Andre Thevenet.
On barber-surgeons, see *The Gory History of Barber-Surgeons; Medieval Medicine Gone Mad* by Aleksa Vuckovic.
On apothecary, see *Herbalist's Charter* by American Botanical Council.
On Henry VIII's apothecary, see *Henry VIII and the Art of Herbal Healing* by PJ Footler.
On dentistry, see *Dental Treatment in Medieval England*, by T Anderson.

Chapter Seven
On the Battle of Agincourt, see *Agincourt; Henry V and the Battle That Made England* by Juliet Barke.
On Fielding Garrison, see *The Face of Mercy* by Matthew Naythons.
On medieval weapons, see *The Weapons of an English Medieval Knight* by M. Cartwright and *The Illustrated History of Knights and the Golden Age of Chivalry* by C. Phillips.
On the Battle of Bosworth and Richard III, see *Bosworth 1485. A Battlefield Rediscovered* by Glenn Foard.
On Ambroise Para, see *Ambroise Pare, A Surgeon in the Field* by James Bruce.
On the Battle of Crecy, see *The Hundred Years War; The English in France 1337–1453* by Desmond Seward.
On the Battle of Hastings and King Harold, see *The Battle of Hastings; The Fall of the Anglo-Saxons and the Rise of the Normans* by Jim Bradbury.
On John Bradmore, see *Great Ideas in the History of Surgery* by Leo Zimmerman.
On Henry V, see *The Disappearing Scar of Henry V* by Anthony Arner, *Agincourt; Henry V and the Battle That Made England* by Juliet Barke, *Saving Prince Hal* by Jo Cummings, and *Prince Hal's Head Wound* by Michael Livingston.
On A Fair Book of Surgery, see *The Surgeon in Medieval English Literature* by Jeremy Citrome.

Chapter Eight

On St Benedict of Nursia and St. Thomas of Canterbury, see *Medieval Monastery* by Mark Cartwright.

On the Hospitallers, see *The Religious Orders in England* by David Knowles.

On Santa Maria of Nuova Hospital France and Hotel Dieu, see *The Ideal Medieval Hospital* by Daniele Cybulskie.

On St. Mary's and St Bartholomew Hospital, see *The Medieval Hospitals of England* by Mary Rotha Clay.

On the Savoy Hospital and Leper hospitals, see *Leprosy in Medieval England* by Carole Rawcliffe and *Medicine and Society in Later Medieval England* by Carole Rawcliffe.

On Praerogativa Regis and King Edward, see *Medieval and Early Renaissance Medicine* by Nancy Saraisi.

On Juanna of Castile, see *Sexuality and Medicine in the Middle Ages* by Danielle Jacquart.

On St. Dymphna of Geel, see, *Asylums and Care for the Insane* by JJ Walsh.

On the Dissolution of the Monasteries and Thomas Cromwell, see *English Monks and the Suppression of the Monasteries* by Geoffrey Baskerville.

Chapter Nine

On Anne Boleyn and the Tower of London, see *Tower, an Epic History of the Tower of London* by Nigel Jones.

On medieval torture methods, see *The Thief, the Cross, and Wheel; Pain and Spectacle of Punishment in Medieval and Renaissance Europe* by Mitchell Merbeck.

On Mary Tudor, see *Fires of Faith: Catholic England Under Mary Tudor* by Eamon Duffy.

On Mary Queen of Scots, see *The Betrayal of Mary, Queen of Scots; Elizabeth I and Her Greatest Rival* by Kate Williams.

On Henry Duke of Cornwall, see *Death Medieval Royal Babies of England* by Cynthia Hugo.

On Purgatory, see *The Birth of Purgatory* by Jacques Le Goff.

On Embalming and the Funeral of Elizabeth of York, Funeral of Henry VIII and Funeral Rites of the Catholic Church, see *Life and Death in the Middle Ages* by Jack Hartnell.

On the Knight's Templar, see *The Persecution of the Knights Templar* by Alain Dumurger and *The Templars* by Dan Jones.

Bibliography

American Botanical Council, 'Herbalist's Charter', *HerbalGram* (1998).
Anderson, T., 'Dental Treatment in Medieval England', *British Dental Journal* (2004).
Arner, Timothy D., 'The Disappearing Scar of Henry V', *Journal of Medieval and Early Modern Studies* (2019).
Barkai, Ron, *A History of Jewish Gynaecological Texts in the Middle Ages* (Brill, 1998).
Barker, Juliet, *Agincourt; Henry V and the Battle That Made England* (New York: Buy Back Books, 2005).
Baskerville, Geoffrey, *English Monks and the Suppression of the Monasteries* (New Haven: Yale University Press, 1937).
Beasley, Brett, *Bad Air; Pollution, Sin and Science Fiction* (Public Domain, 2015).
Beck, Theodore, Richard, *Cutting Edge; Early History of the Surgeons of London* (Lund Humphries, 1974).
Bendick, Jeanne, *Galen-And the Gateway to Medicine* (San Francisco: Ignatius Press, 2002).
Benedicto, Ole Jorgen, *Black Death: The Complete History* (2004).
Billier, PA, *Birth Control in the West in the Thirteenth and Fourteenth Centuries* (1982).
Boccaccio, Giovanni, 'Medical Sourcebook: The Decameron', *Fordham University* (1996).
Bray, RS, *Armies of Pestilence* (New York: Barnes & Noble Books, 1996).
Brown, Kevin, *The Pox-The Life and Near Death of a Very Social Disease* (Stroud, 2006).
Bruce, James, *Ambroise Pare: A Surgeon in the Field* (New York: Viking Penguin, 1981).
Bryson, Sarah, 'The Physical Decline of Henry VIII', The Tudor Society.com, (2016).
Buklijas, Tatjana, 'Croatian Medical Journal', *Medicine and Society in the Medieval Hospital* (2008).
Byrne, Joseph Patrick, *Daily Life during the Black Death* (Greenwood Publishing Group, 2006).
Caballero-Navas, Carmen, *The Book of Women's Love and Jewish Medieval Medical Literature on Women* (Paul Keegan, 2004).
Cantor, N.F., *In the Wake of the Plague* (New York: Free Press, 2001).

Cartwright, M., 'The Weapons of an English Medieval Knight', *Ancient History Encyclopedia* (2018).
Cartwright, Mark, 'Medieval Monastery', *Ancient History Encyclopedia* (2018).
Citrome, Jeremy, *The Surgeon in Medieval English Literature* (New York: Palgrave MacMillan, 2006).
Clay, Rotha Mary, *The Medieval Hospitals of England* (London, 1909).
Cohn-Haft, Louis, *The Public Physicians of Ancient Greece* (Northampton, 1956).
Crawford, Sally, *Childhood in Anglo-Saxon England* (Stroud: Alan Sutton, 1999).
Cummins Jo, 'Saving Prince Hal', *Henry Noble History of Dentistry Research Group*
Cybulskie, Daniele, 'The Ideal Medieval Hospital', Medievalists.net, (2016).
Demurger, Alain, *The Persecution of the Knights Templar* (New York: Pegasus Books, 2019)
Dickens, AG., *The English Reformation* (London: Batsford, 1989).
'Dr William Butts Royal Physician', The Freelance History Writer, (2018).
Duffy, Eamon, *English People and Their Prayers 1240–1570* (New Haven: Yale University Press, 2006).
Eknoyan, Garabed, 'Looking at the Urine; Renaissance of an Unbroken Tradition', *American Journal of Kidney Diseases* (2007).
Fitzharris, Lindsey, 'Behind the Mask; The Plague Doctor', *The Chirurgeons Apprentice* (2014).
Foard, Glenn, *Bosworth, 1485. A Battlefield Rediscovered* (Oxford: Oxbow Books, 2013).
Fondazione IRCCS Ca' Granda Ospedale Maggiore Policlinico https://www.policlinico.mi.it/
Footler, PJ., 'Henry VIII and the Art of Herbal Healing', *The Pharmaceutical Journal* (2009).
Gairdner, James, *The Historical Collections of a Citizen of London in the Fifteen Century* (London, 1876).
Getz, Faye, *Medicine in the English Middle Ages* (Princeton: Princeton University Press, 1998).
Ghosh, Sanjib, 'Henri de Mondeville', *European Journal of Anatomy* (2015).
Gies, J., *Life in a Medieval Castle* (Harper Perennial, 2015).
Given-Wilson, Chris, *An Illustrated History of Late Medieval England* (Manchester: Manchester University Press, 1996).
Gottfried, RS, *The Black Death* (New York: Free Press, 1983).
Green, Monica, *The Trotula: An English Translation of the Medieval Compendium of Women's Medicine* (University of Pennsylvania Press, 2010).
Hanawalt, Barbara, *Growing Up in Medieval London* (New York: Oxford University Press, 1993).
Harthan, John, *The Book of Hours* (New York: Crowell, 1977).
Hutchinson, Robert, *Young Henry: The Rise of Henry VIII* (London: Phoenix Press, 2011).
Hyno, Cynthia, *Medieval Royal Babies of England* (2109).

Jacquart, Danielle, *Sexuality and Medicine in the Middle Ages* (Princeton: Princeton University Press, 1988).
Jones, Dan, *The Templars* (New York: Viking, 2017)
Jones, Peter Murray, 'Performative Rituals for Conception and Childbirth in England',
Jones, WHS, *Philosophy and Medicine in Ancient Greece* (Baltimore: Johns Hopkins Press, 1946).
Katinis, Teodoro, *Medicina e filosofia in Marsilio Ficino: Il Consiglio contra la Pestilentia*. (Rome, 2007).
Kelly, John, *The Great Mortality* (New York: Harper Collins, 2005).
Kirkpatrick, JJ, *Annals of the Royal College of Surgeons in England* (1997).
—. *The Qualities and Conduct of an English Surgeon* (1997).
Knowles, David, *The Religious Orders in England* (Cambridge: Cambridge University Press, 1959).
Knysh, Alexander, *Ibn Arabi in the Later Islamic Tradition* (Suny Press, 1999).
Lang, SJ, *Oxford Dictionary of National Biography-John Bradmore* (Oxford University Press, 2004).
Liebson, Philip, 'The Sweating Sickness in Tudor England; a Plague of the Renaissance', *A Journal of Medical Humanities* (2013).
Livingston, Michael, 'Prince Hal's Head Wound', Medievalist.net, (2013).
Longrigg, James, *Greek Medicine From the Heroic to the Hellenistic Age* (New York, 1998).
Lyons, Jonathan, *The House of Wisdom; How the Arabs Transformed Western Civilization* (Bloomsbury Publishing, 2011).
MacKenzie, Debora, 'Columbus Blamed for Spread of Syphilis', *New Scientist* (2008).
MacRae, Meghan. 'Medieval and Renaissance Depictions of Possession and Exorcism,' *CVLTNation* (2016).
Mason, Stephen, *A History of the Sciences* (New York: Collier Books, 1956).
'Medical Astrology', Medievalastrologyguide.com.
Merback, Mitchell B., *The Thief, the Cross and the Wheel; Pain and the Spectacle of Punishment in Medieval and Renaissance Europe* (London: Reaktion Books, 1999).
Mortimer, Ian, *The Fears of Henry IV* (London: Random House, 2007).
—. *The Time Traveler's Guide to Medieval England* (New York: Simon & Schuster, 2008).
Naythons, Mathew, *The Face of Mercy* (New York: Random House, 1993).
Newman, Simon, 'Religion in the Middle Ages', *The Finer Times* (2008).
Nikiforuk, A., *The Fourth Horseman* (New York: M. Evans and Co., 1993).
Philips, C., *The Illustrated History of Knights & The Golden Age of Chivalry* (Lorenz Books, 2014).
Porter, Roy, *The Greatest Benefit to Mankind: A Medical History of Humanity* (New York: WW Norton, 1997).

Potter, David Stone, *Life Death and Entertainment in the Roman Empire* (University of Michigan Press, 1999).
Powell, Hilary, 'The Miracle of Childbirth: The Portrayal of Parturient Women in Medieval Miracle Narratives', *Social History of Medicine* (2012).
Prescott, Elizabeth, *The English Medieval Hospital* (Melksham: The Cromwell Press Limited, 1992).
Prioreschi, Plinio, *A History of Medicine; Medieval Medicine* (Horatius Press, 1996).
Radcliff, Walter, *Milestones in Midwifery and the Secret Instrument* (Norman Publishing)
Rawcliffe, Carol, *Sources for the History of Medicine in Late Medieval England* (Kalamazoo: Medieval Institute Publications, 1995).
Rawcliffe, Carole, *Leprosy in Medieval England* (Boydell Press, 2016).
—. *Medicine & Society in Later Medieval England* (Gloucestershire: Alan Sutton Publishing, 1995).
Regione Lombardia https://www.asst-settelaghi.it/
Rideal, Rebecca, 'Leprosy and Plague in St. Giles in the Fields', Medievalists.net, (2017).
Risse, Guenter, *Mending Bodies, Saving Souls* (New York: Oxford University Press, 1999).
Roffey, Simon, 'Investigation of a Medieval Pilgrim Burial Excavated from the Leprosarium of St. Mary Magdalen', *Neglected Tropical Diseases* (2017).
—. 'Medieval Leper Hospitals in England; An Archaeological Perspective', *Society for Medieval Archaeology* (2012).
Rosenhek, Jackie, 'Doctors of the Black Death', *Doctor's Review* (2011).
Rowland, Beryl, *Medieval Woman's Guide to Health* (Kent: The Kent State University Press, 1981).
Saraisi, Nancy G., *Medieval & Early Renaissance Medicine* (Chicago: The University of Chicago Press, 1990).
Scarry, Elaine, *The Body in Pain; The Making and Unmaking of the World* (Oxford: Oxford University Press, 1985).
'Secrets Behind the Creepy Plague Doctor Mask and Costume', Ancientorigins.com, (2019).
Sim, A., *A Tudor Housewife* (2010).
Simkin, John, 'Norman Monasteries', *Spartacus Education* (1997).
Slade, Paul, 'The Black Death', Planetslade.com, (2013).
Sterner, Carl, 'A Brief History of Miasmic Theory', *Bulletin of the History of Medicine* (1948).
Thevenet, Andre, 'Guy de Chauliac; The Father of Surgery', *Annals of Vascular Surgery* (1993).
Thomas, Duncan P., *Thomas Vicary and the Anatomie of Mans Body* (2006).
Thurley, S., *Royal Palaces of Tudor England* (1993).
Tracy, Larissa, *Wounds and Wound Repair in Medieval Culture* (Brill, 2015).

Trueman, CN., 'The Lifestyle of Medieval Peasants', HistoryLearningsite.co.uk, (2015).
'Urine Color; Symptoms and Causes', Mayo Clinic (2019).
Vanneste, Sarah Frances, *The Black Death and the Future of Medicine* (Wayne: Wayne State University Press, 2010).
Vuckovic, Aleksa, 'The Gory History of Barber-Surgeons; Medieval Medicine Gone Mad', *Ancient Origins* (2019).
Walsh, J.J., *Asylums and Care for the Insane* (New York: Robert Appleton Company, 1910).
Wayne, Gary, 'What Was Dental Health Like in the Middle Ages', *Dr Gary Wayne Oral and Maxillofacial Surgery* (2015).
Wee, John, 'Discovery of the Zodiac Man in Cuneiform', JSTOR (2015).
Winslow, Charles Edward Amory, *The Conquest of Epidemic Disease* (University of Wisconsin Press, 1980).
Wray, Shona Kelly, 'Children During the Black Death', *Children & Youth in History* (2019).
Zeigler, Philip, *The Black Death* (Harper Collins, 1969).
Zimmerman, Leo, *Great Ideas in the History of Surgery* (Norman Publishing, 2003).
Zuk, Marlene, 'A Great Pox's Greatest Feat; Staying Alive', *New York Times* (2008).